T0304683

Advanced ENT MCQs

Providing over 400 high quality MCQs in the style of the Part 1 FRCS (ORL-HNS) together with clear explanations of not only the correct answer but also a structured way of approaching questions, this revision guide enables exam candidates to prepare for the FRCS (ORL-HNS) Section 1 exam with confidence.

The questions and answers reflect the new approach to the exam and its focus on higher-order judgement and testing real-world clinical decision making. Questions are presented as a common stem with five possible answers, one of which will be the most correct answer: a 'single best answer'. The stem is carefully written, so that every word should help guide candidates to the correct answer. None of the answers will be obviously wrong or dangerous. The candidate must recognise that a 'single best answer' is not the same as a 'single correct answer'. In many of the questions, all the presented answers could be considered correct, but the candidate must choose the best or most appropriate answer from those available.

This book was written by an expert author team who have provided valuable insights and expert content to ensure the book's authority. The content is suitable for exam candidates from the UK and for International ENT trainees preparing to sit the FRCS (ORL-HNS) exam. It is also applicable for candidates preparing for the DOHNS/MRCS ENT exam.

MasterPass Series

Clinical Consultation Skills in Medicine: A Primer for MRCP PACES
Ernest Suresh

Refraction and Retinoscopy: How to Pass the Refraction Certificate, 2E
Jonathan Park, Leo Feinberg, David Jones

The Final FRCA Constructed Response Questions: A Practical Study Guide, 2E
Elizabeth Combeer, Mitul Patel

Diagnostic EMQs: A Comprehensive Collection for Medical Examinations
*Syed Hussain, Umber Rind, Jawed Noori, Yasmean Kalam,
Haseeb Ata and Emanuel Papageorgiou*

Passing the Final FFICM: High-Yield Facts for the MCQ & OSCE Exams
Muzzammil Ali

Cases in Haematology: For the MLA and PLAB
Aaron Niblock

Postgraduate Ophthalmology Exam Success
Maneck Nicholson, Anjali Nicholson, Syed Faraaz Hussain

Pass the MRCP (SCE) Neurology Revision Guide
Dhananjay Gupta

Advanced ENT MCQs: Training to Pass the FRCS (ORL-HNS) Part 1
Peter Kullar, Jameel Muzaffar, Joseph Manjaly

For more information about this series please visit: https://www.routledge.com/MasterPass/book-series/
CRCMASPASS

Advanced ENT MCQs

Training to pass the FRCS (ORL-HNS) Part 1

Peter Kullar, Jameel Muzaffar,
Joseph Manjaly

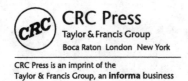

CRC Press
Taylor & Francis Group
Boca Raton London New York

CRC Press is an imprint of the
Taylor & Francis Group, an **informa** business

Designed cover image: AzmanJaka / Getty Images

First edition published 2025
by CRC Press
2385 NW Executive Center Drive, Suite 320, Boca Raton FL 33431

and by CRC Press
4 Park Square, Milton Park, Abingdon, Oxon, OX14 4RN

CRC Press is an imprint of Taylor & Francis Group, LLC

© 2025 Peter Kullar, Jameel Muzaffar and Joseph Manjaly

ISBN: 978-1-032-59519-1
ISBN: 978-1-032-58518-5
ISBN: 978-1-003-45505-9

DOI: 10.1201/9781003455059

Typeset in Century Gothic Pro
by Apex CoVantage, LLC

For Kirsty, Max and Cassia. May the warmth and spirit of California stay with us always.
Peter Kullar

To my wife and family—your patience never fails to surprise me.
Jameel Muzaffar

For Sarah, Joshua and Rosa. Thank you for keeping me going X.
Joseph Manjaly

Books by the same Authors

Advanced ENT Training: A Guide to Passing the FRCS (ORL-HNS) Examination
  ISBN 9780367202514

ENT OSCEs: A Guide to Your First ENT Job and Passing the MRCS (ENT) OSCE
  ISBN 9781032191737

ENT Vivas: A Guide to Passing the Intercollegiate FRCS (ORL-HNS) Viva Examination
  ISBN 9781032113401

Contents

Foreword   xi
About the Authors   xiii
Section Editors   xv
Major Contributors   xvii
Introduction   xix

CHAPTER 1: OTOLOGY   **1**

CHAPTER 2: HEAD AND NECK   **51**

CHAPTER 3: PAEDIATRICS   **87**

CHAPTER 4: RHINOLOGY AND FACIAL PLASTIC SURGERY   **123**

**CHAPTER 5: EVIDENCE-BASED MEDICINE, STATISTICS AND
MISCELLANEOUS**   **167**

INDEX   *181*

Foreword

I remember sitting my FRCS examinations as if they were yesterday; the endless hours of preparation while my young daughter pressed her face up against the window of my study, the exhaustion of having to hit the books after a long day at work and the fear that this may all need to be repeated six months later with a new-born in tow, given the relatively high failure rate. It was something I wanted to be sure that I only had to endure once. Whilst accustomed to sitting exams throughout our training, the stakes are never higher than for the FRCS, which comes at a time when many candidates are already heavily committed both at work, in research and with caring roles within the family, be that for children or other relatives. Those who fail seldom do so because of lack of knowledge and experience, but more often because of poor exam technique. It is therefore critical to be able to access tools to assist with this.

The authors of this textbook build on their success from previous books covering all stages of ENT formative assessment and now complete their series with this guide to passing the MCQ section of the FRCS. Selecting the 'single best answer' involves more than just knowledge, but careful evaluation of both the question and the possible answers in order to make a value judgement as to the best fit. This needs practice to perfect. The text provides an excellent opportunity to do so with questions covering the full breadth of the syllabus with clear explanations supporting the 'most correct' answer. This will be an invaluable resource for anyone sitting the FRCS(ORLHNS)—I certainly wish their books had been available in my day.

Reviews of their previous books demonstrate the commitment of the authors, Peter Kullar, Jameel Muzaffar and Joseph Manjaly, to medical education and supporting those that follow in their footsteps. They have assembled a formidable team of senior trainees and young consultants to assist them in producing this volume, for which the five star reviews will quickly follow. It's a great privilege to be asked to introduce this book, and I'd like to take the opportunity to congratulate all the authors, and to thank them on behalf of all those preparing for their FRCS exams who will benefit.

Professor Claire Hopkins
MA (Oxon), BMBCh, FRCS(ORLHNS), DM
Professor of Rhinology
Guy's and St Thomas' NHS Hospitals Trust, UK

About the Authors

Peter Kullar is a Clinical Instructor in Neurotology/Lateral Skull Base Surgery at Stanford University. He was previously an NIHR academic lecturer and a Wellcome Trust/Royal College of Surgeons clinical research fellow at the University of Cambridge. Peter is the author of two MasterPass series books *Advanced ENT Training: A Guide to Passing the FRCS (ORL-HNS) Examination* and *ENT OSCEs: A Guide to Your First ENT Job and Passing the MRCS (ENT) OSCE* (one FRCS and one MRCS).

Jameel Muzaffar is Consultant in Otology and Auditory Implantation at University Hospitals Birmingham, Honorary Senior Research Fellow at the University of Birmingham and National Specialty Lead for ENT for the National Institute of Health and Care Research (NIHR) Research Delivery Network. He was previously TWJ Foundation fellow in Otology and Auditory Implantation in Cambridge and prior to that Honorary Royal College of Surgeons research fellow. He remains part of the Sensory Encoding and Neurosensory Engineering (SENSE) Lab, through which he first met Peter Kullar. Jameel is an editor of CRC Press *ENT Vivas: A Guide to Passing the Intercollegiate FRCS (ORL-HNS) Viva Examination* 9781032113401.

Joseph Manjaly is Consultant Otologist, Auditory Implant and ENT surgeon, specialising in ear and hearing problems for adults and children. He is currently clinical lead for adult ENT at the Royal National ENT Hospital and University College London Hospitals, UK. He is a member of the British Society of Otology Council and also produces educational ENT and medical content on social media as @earsurgeonjoe

Section Editors

HEAD AND NECK

Raghav Dwivedi PhD FRCS (ORL-HNS)
Consultant ENT/Head and Neck/Thyroid
    Surgeon
University College London Hospitals NHS
    Foundation Trust
Honorary Associate Professor, Division of
    Surgery and Interventional Science
University College London
London, UK

Jonathan Fussey MBChB MD FRCS
    (ORL-HNS)
Consultant Head and Neck Surgeon
University Hospitals Birmingham NHS
    Foundation Trust
Birmingham, UK

Hannah Nieto BSc MBBS PhD FRCS
    (ORL-HNS)
Clinician Scientist
University of Birmingham
Birmingham, UK

RHINOLOGY

Adnan Darr BSc(Hons) MSc MBChB
    DOHNS PGCME FRCS (ORL-HNS)
Consultant Rhinologist and Anterior Skull
    Base Surgeon
University Hospitals Coventry and
    Warwickshire NHS Foundation Trust
Coventry, UK

Karan Jolly MBChB FRCS (ORL-HNS)
Consultant Rhinologist and Anterior Skull
    Base Surgeon
University Hospitals Birmingham NHS
    Foundation Trust
Birmingham, UK

FACIAL PLASTIC SURGERY

Monica Rossi Meyer MD
Attending Facial Plastic Surgeon
Vanderbilt University Medical Center
Nashville, Tennessee, USA

MISCELLANEOUS AND EVIDENCE-BASED MEDICINE

Baptiste Leurent PhD
Associate Professor in Medical Statistics
Department of Statistical Science
    University College London
London, UK

PAEDIATRICS

Amit Parmar MBBS MSc FRCS (ORL-HNS)
Consultant Paediatric ENT Surgeon
Birmingham Children's Hospital
Birmingham, UK

Major Contributors

HEAD AND NECK

Vikas Acharya BMBS MA MBA FRCS(ORL-HNS) FHEA MAcadMEd MFSTEd
Specialist Registrar (ST8) in Ear, Nose and Throat Surgery
The Royal National ENT Hospital and University College London Hospitals
London, UK

Vikram Padaye MBBS PhD FRACS
Adult and Paediatric Ear, Nose and Throat Surgeon
Sleep Apnoea and Sinus Specialist
University of Adelaide
Adelaide, Australia

RHINOLOGY

Vikas Acharya BMBS MA MBA FRCS (ORL-HNS) FHEA MAcadMEd MFSTEd
Specialist Registrar (ST8) in Ear, Nose and Throat Surgery
The Royal National ENT Hospital and University College London Hospitals
London, UK

Zechariah Franks MD MPH
Senior Associate Consultant
Division of Rhinology, Department of Otolaryngology, Head and Neck Surgery
Mayo Clinic
Jacksonville, Florida, USA

FACIAL PLASTIC SURGERY

Abdul Nassimizadeh MBChB BMedSci FRCS (ORL-HNS)
Locum Consultant Rhinologist and Facial Plastic Surgeon
University Hospitals Birmingham NHS Foundation Trust
Birmingham, UK

MISCELLANEOUS AND EVIDENCE-BASED MEDICINE

Munira Ally MBBS DOHNS MRCS
ENT Specialty Registrar
Lister Hospital
Stevenage, UK

PAEDIATRICS

Munira Ally MBBS DOHNS MRCS
ENT Specialty Registrar
Lister Hospital
Stevenage, UK

Taseer F Din MBChB FCORL MMED
Assistant Professor of Clinical Otolaryngology Head and Neck Surgery
Weill Cornell Medical College, Qatar

OTOLOGY

Cillian Forde BSc (Hons) MB BChir (Cantab) DOHNS FRCS (ORL-HNS)
ENT Specialty Registrar
Royal National ENT Hospital and University College London Hospitals
London, UK

Reshma Ghedia MBBS BSc(Hons) FRCS (ORL-HNS)
Otology and Neurotology Fellow
Queen Elizabeth II Health Sciences Centre, Halifax, Nova Scotia, Canada

Fiona McClenaghan BSc MBBS DOHNS FRCS (ORL-HNS)
Lateral Skull Base Fellow
Guy's and St Thomas' and King's College Hospital London
London, UK

Ankit Patel MBBS BSc Dip (M.Med) FRCS (ORL-HNS)
ENT Specialty Registrar
Royal National ENT Hospital and University College London Hospitals
London, UK

Bhavesh Patel MBBS BSc(Hons) MEd(Surg) DOHNS FRCS (ORL-HNS)
Consultant ENT Surgeon
London Northwest University Healthcare NHS Trust
London, UK

Dalal Sabban MBBS DES-ORLCCF
Otology and Auditory Implant Fellow
Royal National ENT Hospital and University College London Hospitals
London, UK

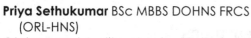

Priya Sethukumar BSc MBBS DOHNS FRCS
  (ORL-HNS)
Otology and Auditory Implant Fellow
Royal National ENT Hospital and
  University College London
  Hospitals
London, UK

Benjamin Silver MBBS BSc MRCS DOHNS
ENT Specialty Registrar
Royal National ENT Hospital and University
  College London Hospitals
London, UK

Elinor Warner MBBS MA(Oxon) PG cert FRCS
  (ORL-HNS)
ENT Specialty Registrar Royal National
ENT Hospital & University College London
  Hospitals
London, UK

Introduction

The Intercollegiate Specialty Fellowship exam, more commonly known simply as the 'FRCS', represents a significant milestone on the way to obtaining a Certificate of Completion of Training (CCT) or Certificate of Eligibility for Specialist Registration (CESR) and becoming a consultant surgeon in the United Kingdom.

The exam is divided into two parts: Section 1, often called 'the MCQ' or 'the written' and Section 2, typically referred to as 'the viva and clinicals'. Section 1 is often seen, somewhat unfairly, as a warm-up for the more important and rigorous Section 2. However, whilst Section 2 has several high-quality resources available, candidates have, in years previous, struggled to find resources targeted at the latest iteration of Section 1. The scope of the exam is huge, covering the breadth of ENT and allied specialities and therefore the importance of exam-specific revision cannot be over-emphasised. Our intention was to create a book that made preparing for the exam a little easier and less daunting for candidates across the UK and around the world.

In previous generations, Section 1 focussed on straight factual recall, and whilst the questions may have been hard, particularly if they explored an area of hazy knowledge, there was little confusion as to what the question was asking. More recently, the examiners' approach has changed, focussing on higher-order judgement, and testing real-world clinical decision making.

Questions are presented as a common stem with five possible answers, one of which will be the *most* correct answer: a 'single best answer'. The stem is carefully designed to not contain extraneous information, so every word should help guide candidates to the correct answer. None of the answers will be obviously wrong or dangerous. The candidate must recognise that a 'single best answer' is not the same as a 'single correct answer'. In many of the questions, all the presented answers could be considered correct, but the candidate must choose the best or most appropriate answer from those available. The highest-performing questions, those that discriminate between candidates at the pass/fail boundary, often test multi-logical thinking whereby multiple pieces of knowledge must be systematically applied to solve a problem. Nevertheless, it should be remembered that if a question looks easy, then it probably is, and the examiners are generally not trying to trick the candidates. These changes in question setting style have accompanied an update of core topics, which now include newer relevant topics such as immunotherapy and hearing preservation cochlear implantation.

It is important to read the wording of the questions carefully. For example, a question asking for the 'best *first* treatment' may have a different answer from one asking for the 'best *definitive* treatment'. Questions exploring anatomy and physiology are integrated into clinical scenarios, rather than being presented as direct factual recall, and there will be far fewer 'name the syndrome' style questions, though of course the underlying knowledge remains of use. Whilst the aim of this approach to testing performance is laudable, it can be particularly stressful for candidates, when multiple answers are presented and most sound as though they could be correct. We would encourage candidates to not be paralysed by uncertainty. Due to these subtleties, many questions prove not to be clear discriminators between candidates and are removed from the examination. Rest assured there is extensive standard setting that happens behind the scenes that ensures the exam is a valid assessment of the curriculum and can distinguish between good and poorly performing candidates.

Candidates must realise that time is of the essence in the exam, and it is important to move quickly through the questions without dwelling on those you find difficult. If you are genuinely unsure, make a choice, 'flag' the question and move on. If time remains at the end of the examination, you can always return to your flagged questions and think again. There is no negative marking, so it is imperative that you answer every question.

As with other books in this series, the content has been written by early-stage consultants, post-CCT fellows or exceptional registrars near the end of training. We have gratefully received contributions from colleagues around the country and our team of senior editors have both provided invaluable insights and ensured the book's authority.

We, as your authors, set out to create this book with the explicit aim of giving candidates access to high-quality questions in the style of the Section 1 examination, with clear explanations of not only the correct answer but also a structured way of approaching questions that can be applied to other topics in the exam. This is the book we would have valued most in the run up to our own examinations and we hope you find it helpful. Preparing for the FRCS (ORL-HNS) is a tough journey both for you and those around you, but if we have written a book that provides candidates with a more realistic understanding of what the exam entails and guides your revision appropriately then we have achieved what we set out to do. If you have suggestions to improve the book, or ideas for other topics that you would like to see us cover, we would be grateful for your thoughts.

It also brings us personal joy that this book completes a series of UK ENT exam textbooks that now guides doctors through all of the required hurdles from first ENT job to starting as a consultant—a generational contribution we hope has helped many!

Peter Kullar, Jameel Muzaffar and Joseph Manjaly

CHAPTER 1: OTOLOGY

1. **A 36-year-old male has a subtotal petrosectomy and blind sac closure surgery for clearance of extensive unilateral recurrent cholesteatoma. He now has a unilateral mixed hearing loss with bone conduction thresholds of 50dB. He is keen for help as soon as possible to reduce the functional impact of single-sided deafness. Which is the optimal hearing rehabilitation option?**
   A Conventional hearing aid
   B Ossiculoplasty
   C Percutaneous bone-anchored hearing implant
   D OSIA transcutaneous bone conduction hearing implant
   E Bonebridge transcutaneous bone conduction hearing implant

2. **A 23-year-old patient presents with pulsatile tinnitus that is not in synchrony with the patient's heartbeat. The most likely diagnosis is:**
   A Intracranial hypertension
   B Atherosclerosis
   C Arteriovenous malformation
   D Paraganglioma
   E Palatal myoclonus

3. **The following is the most important prognostic consideration when attempting to restore sound localisation to an 18-year-old with unilateral profound hearing loss and normal contralateral hearing:**
   A Number of hours per day wearing a CROS aid
   B Number of hours per day using a bone conduction implant
   C Duration of deafness

   D Status of the ipsilateral vestibulocochlear nerve
   E Status of the contralateral vestibulocochlear nerve

4. **You are performing a combined approach tympanomastoidectomy for an extensive cholesteatoma. During malleus removal, a tendon is divided that was inserted into the malleus neck. Lying more medial to the tendon origin point, and immediately superior, a structure is revealed due to the extent of bone erosion caused by the cholesteatoma. This structure is likely:**
   A The cog
   B The supratubal recess
   C The geniculate ganglion
   D The oval window
   E The malleus head

5. **A 55-year-old man presents with a 3-month history of increasing right-sided otalgia and otorrhoea. He has been treated with repeated microsuction and topical antibiotics. Despite this the discharge is worsening and his sleep is disturbed by pain. Bloodwork shows normal white cell count and C-reactive protein. Which is most significant in determining the diagnosis?**
   A A history of radiotherapy for nasopharyngeal carcinoma
   B CT temporal bones showing bony erosion of the external auditory canal
   C Microbiology demonstrating growth of pseudomonas
   D Non-echoplanar diffusion-weighted MRI
   E Technetium 99 bone scan

DOI: 10.1201/9781003455059-1

6. **A patient coughs whilst having ear wax removed by microsuction. Which nerve is responsible for this?**

   A Trigeminal nerve

   B Facial nerve

   C Jacobson's nerve

   D Glossopharyngeal nerve

   E Arnold's nerve

7. **Cochlear implantation aims to stimulate the spiral ganglion cells, composed of axons derived from the cochlear nerve. These axons, as well as the cochlear blood supply, both run through the length of which structure?**

   A Helicotrema

   B Stria vascularis

   C Modiolus

   D Reissner's membrane

   E Organ of Corti

8. **A patient's ability to localise sound is compromised with mild hearing loss. In addition to hearing level asymmetry, which other factor is most likely to be implicated?**

   A Pinna shape

   B Reduced intelligence quotient

   C Presence of bilateral middle ear effusion

   D Presence of an intact vestibulo-ocular reflex

   E Presence of intact stapedial reflexes

9. **A 55-year-old patient with previously normal hearing presents four days after developing left-sided hearing loss after an upper respiratory tract infection. Weber tuning fork test lateralised to the right, Rinne is positive bilaterally and an audiogram shows an asymmetry of masked bone conduction thresholds. There is an ongoing medical history inclusive of peptic ulcer disease and poorly controlled diabetes. Which is the most appropriate initial management?**

   A Prednisolone 1 mg/kg orally once per day for 7 days

   B Prednisolone 0.5 mg/kg orally once per day for 7 days followed by gradual weaning of the dose over the following 10 days

   C Dexamethasone 0.2 mg/kg orally once per day for 7 days

   D Methylprednisolone 62.5 mg/ml intra-tympanic injection

   E Dexamethasone 0.2 mg/ml intratympanic injection

10. **You perform tympanomastoid surgery for a 20-year-old female with cholesteatoma. The facial nerve is noted to be dehiscent intra-operatively and the facial nerve monitor activates during the procedure. Scratch test is normal post-operatively. On Day 3 the patient develops a new-onset ipsilateral grade 6 facial palsy. What is the first appropriate management step?**

    A Tympanomastoid re-exploration

    B CT temporal bone scan

    C Prednisolone 1 mg/kg OD

    D Methylprednisolone 62.5 mg/ml intra-tympanic injection

    E MRI brain and internal auditory canals with contrast

11. **A 65-year-old patient with stage 4 laryngeal cancer undergoes surgery and postoperative radiotherapy and chemotherapy. She has had one round of IV chemotherapy and subsequently noticed right-sided tinnitus. She had no previous hearing loss or tinnitus. Her oncologist contacts you for advice about her next dose which is planned for tomorrow:**

    A Continue with cisplatin chemotherapy and provide oral steroid cover

    B Continue with cisplatin chemotherapy and offer transtympanic steroid injection

C Continue with cisplatin chemotherapy and offer transtympanic sodium
thiosulphate injection
D Advise to hold cisplatin chemotherapy and conduct a hearing test
E Advise to prescribe hyperbaric oxygen

12. **A 40-year-old patient who had a recent
admission with urosepsis attends your
clinic with recurrent falls and hearing
loss. She said the world keeps moving.
She said she had blood tests during the
hospitalisation that confirmed the antibiotic was in the therapeutic range. She
has a family history of hearing loss. Her
hearing test confirms bilateral severe
sensorineural hearing loss and her
head thrust test is positive bilaterally.
Which test would be the most useful?**
A MRI
B Caloric testing
C vHIT
D Genetic testing
E Rotatory chair testing and
posturography

13. **A 46-year-old patient attends with
hearing loss on the left side which
occurred gradually during the time he
has been working at a printing press.
A request to be seen has been made by**

occupational health at his workplace.
He denies any other otological symp-
toms or previous infections or surgery.
On examination there are no significant
findings. The audiogram is shown below.
What is the best test you can organise to
confirm his hearing loss? (See Figure 1.1)
A Request an MRI internal auditory
meati (MRI IAM)
B Request cortical evoked response
audiometry
C Request speech audiometry
D Request auditory brainstem response
testing
E Request otoacoustic emission testing

14. **A 46-year-old patient attends with
hearing loss on the left side which
occurred gradually during the time he
has been working at a printing press.
A request to be seen has been made
by occupational health at his work. He
denies any other otological symptoms
or previous infections or surgery. On
examination there are no significant
findings. You are handed his hearing
test which he had just before seeing
you. The audiogram is shown below.
Which test result will you prioritise?**
A Pure tone audiogram
B Tympanogram

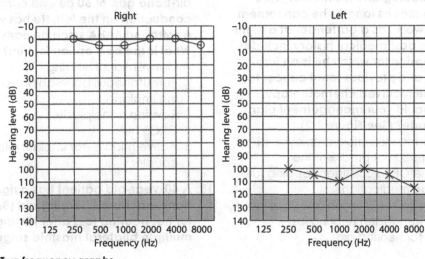

Figure 1.1 Two frequency graphs.

C Stapedial reflexes

D Word recognition score (WRS)

E Speech recognition threshold (SRT)

15. **A 13-year-old who has never had any previous medical issues attends your clinic with his mother. Mum explains that he says he cannot hear and has been performing very poorly at school and requires a lot of help. Mum reports that he refuses to go to school sometimes because he cannot hear the teachers and she often has to stay at home with him. The audiologist attempted to perform a hearing test today but said there was poor test reliability with inconsistent responses. There are type A tympanograms on both sides. The child spoke with normal speech but very infrequently and examination was normal. Which test could you perform today to help create your management plan?**

   A Distortion product OAE

   B Auditory brainstem responses

   C Cortical evoked response audiometry

   D Speech audiometry

   E Stapedial reflexes

16. **A 42-year-old presents with bilateral sensorineural hearing loss and the following audiogram. His mother wore hearing aids as long as he can remember. He works as a bartender at a nightclub. His past medical history includes hypertension for which he is on furosemide and previous renal cancer for which he received chemotherapy. What should your management plan not include? (See Figure 1.2)**

   A Consider alternative employment

   B Prescription of prednisolone

   C Ask the GP to consider stopping furosemide medication

   D Ensure he seeks urgent medical input if he has sudden hearing loss

   E Refer for hearing aids

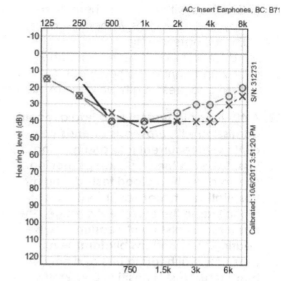

Figure 1.2 Hearing graph.

17. **A 20-year-old who had failed atresiaplasty for congenital ear canal atresia when he was younger would like a second opinion about his hearing rehabilitation. On examination he has a slightly smaller right ear with evidence of a complete ear canal stenosis. His left ear is normal. He has had a CT scan. He works in an office but plays football in a local league which he is passionate about. His hearing test confirms normal bone conduction on the right with an air-bone gap of 60 dB and normal air conduction on the left. He has worn a softband BAHA since an early age. What is the best option for him?**

   A Conventional hearing aid

   B Percutaneous bone-anchored hearing implant

   C Revision canalplasty

   D CROS aid

   E Active middle-ear implant with stapes coupler

18. **A 40-year-old patient has a right bone-anchored hearing aid (BAHA) for her hearing loss after having had multiple bilateral mastoid surgeries**

many years ago. She works as a secretary and explains that the BAHA has significantly improved her quality of life. However, in the last year she has seen you frequently for crusting and discharge and can now no longer place the processor on top because of skin growing over it. She is struggling at work and is worried about losing her job so wants something to be done as soon as possible. What is the best option for her?

A Revise the skin around the BAHA

B Replace with a longer abutment

C Insert a new BAHA at a separate site

D Use a BAHA on a softband

E Offer an implantable device

19. **A 40-year-old man presented with left-sided gradual hearing loss for which he had an MRI internal auditory meati (MRI IAM) with contrast which shows an intracanalicular vestibular schwannoma. His audiogram confirms a left-sided sensorineural hearing loss reaching 45 dB in the higher frequencies and normal hearing on the right side. He has tried a behind-the-ear hearing aid on that side but reports that the noise is garbled. What test could you do to ascertain why this is the cause?**

A Speech recognition threshold

B Word recognition score

C Repeat MRI

D Speech in noise test

E Repeat audiogram

20. **A 72-year-old patient with severe rheumatoid arthritis attends with bilateral downsloping severe high-frequency sensorineural hearing loss. She previously had hearing aids which worked well but she stopped using them because she has issues with her voice feeling "boomy". She has no prior otological history or risk factors. Examination showed narrow canals but**

free of wax. Which hearing aid would be best?

A Behind the ear with a custom mould

B Behind the ear with an open fit dome

C A receiver-in-the-ear (RITE) aid

D In-the-ear (ITE) aid

E In-the-canal (ITC) aid

21. **A 75-year-old man has bilateral downsloping hearing loss. He explains that his friend, who is 50 years old and has nearly identical hearing loss to his audiogram, gave him his hearing aids to try but they don't work for him, and the sound is distorted. What is the reason for this?**

A Loudness recruitment

B Paracusis of Willis

C Cocktail party effect

D Binaural squelch

E Neural presbycusis

22. **A 60-year-old has been referred with recurrent bilateral ear itching and discharge on both sides. She has no other medical issues. On examination you remove her in-the-canal hearing aids to reveal that she has erythema and scaling at the external meatus but the medial ear canal and drum are otherwise normal. How would you manage this?**

A Prescribe steroid ointment

B Refer for an allergy test

C Refer to the audiologist to create ventilation holes in her ear moulds

D Refer for a bone-anchored hearing aid

E Treat with Sofradex drops

23. **You are seeing a 16-year-old boy in your clinic with his parents. He was admitted in hospital for a week with bacterial meningitis. Five days into his admission he reported having bilateral hearing loss. He started prednisolone 60mg on the same day which he finished yesterday. He says he has not noticed an improvement in his hearing. His hearing test confirms bilateral**

profound sensorineural hearing loss. What is the best definitive course of action?

A 1 week more of prednisolone 60 mg
B Bilateral transtympanic steroid injections
C Referral for conventional hearing aids
D Urgent referral for a cochlear implant assessment
E Order a CT scan

24. A child was born two weeks ago after a normal vaginal delivery to healthy parents. After birth he failed automated otoacoustic emissions (AOAE) whilst in hospital. He attended a new appointment with his parents and had clear responses for AOAE when repeated. Mum explained that she had noticed that he has a bifid uvula. What is the next course of action?

A Discharge them and advise them to monitor their child's development
B Refer for immediate audiological assessment
C Refer for audiological assessment to take place at 7 to 9 months of age
D Refer for automated auditory brainstem response
E Repeat AOAE

25. A 62-year-old male presents with a bilateral symmetrical downsloping hearing loss reaching 80 dB, tinnitus and imbalance without a rotatory component. His word recognition score is 60% on both sides at 100 dB. He is on furosemide for his heart failure. His main issue is that he cannot hear well at church. He said that his current hearing aids are not good enough in that setting but work well otherwise. What should he be offered?

A Loop system
B Cochlear implantation
C Frequency modulation or digital modulation system
D Bone-anchored hearing aid

E Bonebridge transcutaneous hearing implant

26. Which of the following medications would be most appropriate for use in the management of otomycosis?

A Sofradex
B Ciloxan
C Ofloxacin
D Locorten Vioform
E Gentisone HC

27. A 42-year-old lady presents with a 3-year history of left-sided muffled hearing but no aural discharge. Audiometry shows a mild left conductive hearing loss (10 dB air-bone gap). Otoscopy shows the following appearance. What is the most appropriate management?

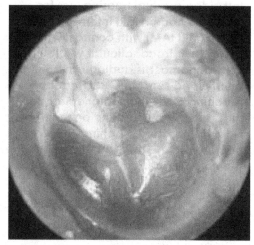

Figure 1.3 Ear drum photo.

A Reassurance and discharge
B Hearing aid assessment and review in 6–12 months
C Ventilation tube placement
D Ossiculoplasty
E Tympanomastoid surgery

28. Which of the following statements is true of otosclerosis?

A It follows an autosomal recessive inheritance pattern
B Foci may originate from the incus
C Otosclerotic bone is denser than natural bone

D It can cause sensorineural hearing loss

E Stapes surgery is always indicated

29. Which of the following is not a potential consequence of an inadequately sized stapes prosthesis?

A Vertigo

B Facial weakness

C Piston migration

D Fluctuating hearing loss

E Permanent hearing loss

30. Which of the following prostheses can be used when there is a mobile footplate but an absent stapes superstructure?

A Total ossicular replacement prosthesis

B Partial ossicular replacement prosthesis

C Footplate prosthesis

D Malleus replacement prosthesis

E Bone cement (Otomimix, Ketac Cem etc.)

31. Which of the following surgeries carries the greatest risk of facial palsy?

A Tympanomastoid surgery for cholesteatoma

B Stapedotomy

C Tympanoplasty

D Ventilation tube placement

E Intratympanic steroids administration

32. Which of the following is not a recognised risk factor for the development of otitis media with effusion in children?

A Craniofacial anomalies

B Parental smoking

C High socioeconomic background

D Attendance at day care facilities

E Bottle-feeding

33. A 35-year-old man presents with a 4-day history of otalgia but no otorrhoea. Otoscopy shows a bulging and erythematous tympanic membrane and examination shows mild tenderness over the mastoid cortex with extensive soft tissue oedema. There is however no erythema. Which eponymous sign is described?

A Griesinger's sign

B Hitselberger's sign

C Brown's sign

D Hennebert's sign

E Tullio phenomenon

34. A 28-year-old woman presents with a 6-day history of progressive otalgia and fever but no otorrhoea. Otoscopy shows a bulging and erythematous tympanic membrane and examination shows some erythema and tenderness over the temporalis muscle. What is described here?

A Citelli's abscess

B Bezold's abscess

C Luc's abscess

D Zygomatic root abscess

E Mastoid abscess

35. Under which of the following circumstances would a blind sac closure be an appropriate option?

A Primary tympanomastoid surgery for cholesteatoma confined to the middle ear and antrum and a mild-moderate CHL

B Second revision surgery following an ear canal wall down procedure with extensive cholesteatoma and a large conductive hearing loss

C Primary tympanomastoid surgery for extensive cholesteatoma with erosion of the ossicular chain

D Revision surgery for a small mesotympanic recurrence but with a 10 dB air-bone gap

E Second revision surgery with an intact posterior ear canal wall and a recurrence in the epitympanum

36. A first-time mother seeks input for her 8-month-old daughter who doesn't turn when called. Examination shows a peanut-shaped pinna on the right and normal ear canal and pinna on the left. There were no other pre- or postnatal concerns. The audiologist informs her that unilateral hearing loss will not impact her speech development. What

would you suggest as the next suitable step?

A Refer to a plastic surgeon for pinna reconstruction now

B Refer to a plastic surgeon for a pinna reconstruction before the child starts school

C Provide the child with an air conduction hearing aid

D Provide the child with a softband bone conduction hearing aid

E Perform aetiological investigations to establish a likely underlying syndromic cause

37. **A 4-year-old with unilateral right-sided microtia has been issued a softband bone conduction hearing aid but is experiencing teasing at school and only wears it for a few hours at home. She has been referred to the auditory implant clinic to discuss options. What is the best initial option for her?**

A Explore ways of overcoming obstacles to softband use

B Right-sided OSIA bone conduction implant

C Canalplasty

D Right-sided Bonebridge bone conduction implant

E Right-sided cochlear implant

38. **A 76-year-old patient with bilateral severe otosclerosis is undergoing assessment for a cochlear implant. An audiogram is performed as part of the assessment. Which one of the following responses is most correct?**

A Masking should be used to reveal the true audiometric thresholds for each ear

B True bone conduction thresholds on the audiogram are likely to be compromised for this patient due to the masking dilemma

C The patient should have a stapedectomy performed and then can be re-assessed for suitability for cochlear implantation

D Cochlear implantation is not an option in this patient due to cochlear otosclerosis

E The audiogram is likely to show a sensorineural hearing loss pattern

39. **A 14-year-old girl has combined-approach tympanoplasty for cholesteatoma in her only hearing ear. Pre-operatively she had been getting vertigo with loud noises and during microsuction. During the surgery when elevating the cholesteatoma matrix off the anterior limb of the superior semicircular canal, there is concern about a labyrinthine fistula. What is the best next step in this case?**

A Continue elevating the matrix and cover with temporalis facia, bone dust and fibrin glue

B Stop and leave the matrix over the semi-circular canal and monitor with DWI MRI scanning

C Stop and leave the matrix over the semi-circular canal and plan to return in 3–6 months to remove the matrix

D Laser 100 ms 1 watt to the matrix

E Stop and leave the matrix over the semi-circular canal and obliterate the whole mastoid cavity

40. **A 10-year-old boy with trisomy 21 has had surgery for extensive left-sided cholesteatoma 5 years ago and reconstruction with a TORP ossiculoplasty. He denies recent infections, but his dad is keen for an option to improve his hearing to help him be more independent. He has been issued a softband hearing aid which he wears sometimes when at school. DWI MRI has shown mastoid opacification with no restricted diffusion. Audiogram shows a maximal conductive hearing loss on the left and mild hearing loss on the right with bilateral flat tympanograms. What is the best initial option to try to improve hearing for the patient?**

A Bilateral grommet insertion

B Cochlear OSIA bone conducting implant

C MED-EL Bonebridge implant

D Revision TORP ossiculoplasty

E Encourage softband use

41. A 45-year-old cleaner attends your clinic with a 3-year history of a discharging left ear and hearing loss. Examination shows an attic crust which comes out cleanly when you microsuction the ear to reveal an auto-atticotomy cavity. What is the best definitive option to offer the patient?

A Cartilage tympanoplasty +/- ossiculoplasty

B Combined-approach tympanomastoidectomy

C Instil some trimovate cream and review in clinic in 4 weeks

D Offer an air conduction hearing aid

E Offer a bone conduction hearing aid

42. A 59-year-old male with a history of chemo-radiotherapy treatment 10 years ago for a right-sided T4 maxillary SCC presents with pain and discharge from his right ear which has been ongoing for a few months. This has been treated in primary care with several courses of topical antibiotics but the pain and discharge persist. Examination reveals no lesion but some exposed bone at the floor of the ear canal and microsuction is painful. Swabs reveal a mixed growth. What is the best additional treatment option?

A Biopsy of the ear canal

B Pentoxifylline and vitamin E

C Oral steroids

D Combination topical antibiotic and steroid drops

E Lateral temporal bone resection

43. A 36-year-old man developed right ear pain, headaches and fevers, and was treated with oral antibiotics. After 1 week the ear started discharging but he then developed symptoms in the contralateral ear which continued alongside headaches. He was referred to the urgent referral clinic for microsuction. Cultures from the ear canal grew *Streptococcus pneumoniae*, and examination revealed some ear canal discharge in the right ear and a bulging tympanic membrane on the left. The patient was admitted for IV antibiotics. CT temporal bones showed opacification in both middle ears and some erosion of the temporal bone. MRI scan was performed which revealed a small 2mm epidural abscess on the left side. What is the best definitive treatment option?

A Continue IV antibiotics

B Regular microsuction and topical antibiotics and IV antibiotics

C EUA ears and grommet insertion

D Referral to neurosurgery

E Bilateral cortical mastoidectomies

44. A 24-year-old man is admitted under the neurosurgical team after a road traffic accident sustaining significant head trauma. He had blood coming from his right ear after injury and was intubated at the scene. CT head shows brain contusions and a right temporal bone fracture through the otic capsule. There were reports that there was forehead weakness and difficulty closing the right eye at the scene but the patient is now intubated and ventilated on ITU. What would be your initial investigation approach in this patient?

A Electromyography (EMG) on day 3

B Electroneurography between days 3–21

C Electroneurography after 4 weeks

D Audiogram

E Wait until patient is extubated to re-assess

45. A 34-year-old man is noted to have a positive focus of restricted diffusion on his DWMRI scan one year after combined-approach tympanomastoidectomy. He is listed for revision surgery which is undertaken uneventfully. He is

discharged the same day. A week later he presents to his GP with a red, swollen, itchy, weeping ear and given some oral antibiotics. The post-operative follow-up is expedited, packing is removed and things settle down. He has now developed a cholesteatoma in the other ear. What precautions should be taken at the next surgery?

A Oral antibiotics intra-operatively

B Oral antibiotics for 7 days post-operatively

C An earlier follow-up appointment for removal of packing

D Pope wick and topical ofloxacin used to pack the ear

E No precautions; it is just unlucky

46. A 67-year-old man with type II diabetes developed a painful discharging right ear which has been ongoing for 6 months. Blood tests show a normal white cell count and a raised C-reactive protein (CRP). A CT scan showed erosion of the bony canal wall and the patient was started on oral ciprofloxacin 750 mg BD alongside regular microsuction. The pain and ear canal changes had resolved when seen in clinic. Which is the most useful investigation to determine the end of treatment?

A CRP

B Gallium 67 tagged white blood cell scan

C Technetium 99m bone scan (Tc99m)

D Repeat CT

E Ear swab

47. A 55-year-old hypertensive patient presents with new-onset left-sided hearing loss 5 days after developing an upper respiratory tract infection. He has had no ear pain or discharge but feels a blocked feeling in his left ear. His tuning fork tests are as follows: Weber to the right side. Rinne AC > BC bilaterally. There is no capacity for an audiogram today. What is the most appropriate next step in management?

A MRI IAM

B Intratympanic steroid injections

C Oral steroid course

D Reassurance

E Topical antibiotic/steroid ear drops

48. A 64-year-old presents to your clinic with a 3-day history of severe right-sided hearing loss and imbalance. He has been recently started on insulin by his GP which is failing to control his diabetes and is awaiting an endocrinology follow-up. He also has a history of gastric ulcers. On examination his tympanic membranes are unremarkable. His audiogram confirms a 70 dB right-sided sensorineural hearing loss. No previous audiograms are available for comparison. What is the most reasonable next step in management?

A Oral steroid course + PPI

B Intratympanic steroid injection

C MRI IAM

D Vasculitis/Syphilis/Lyme screen

E Expedite endocrinology follow-up

49. A 60-year-old male presents to the clinic with a right-sided whooshing noise in time with his pulse. He has had this noise present for years, but it is now affecting his sleep. He has no hearing loss. The noise does change with head movements. His ear examination is normal. The noise reduces when you compress the neck on the right side. You do not hear any bruits on auscultation. Which investigation is most useful in this case?

A Pure tone audiogram

B MRI neck/head with contrast – arterial and venous phases

C CT neck/head with contrast – arterial and venous phases (CT A/V)

D High-resolution CT temporal bones

E MRI internal acoustic meatus

50. A 37-year-old female presents to the clinic with right-sided hearing loss and discharge. She describes imbalance when an ambulance drives past and the ability to hear her own voice

echoing in her ear. On examination, she has purulent discharge within the right ear canal and a polyp is occluding the tympanic membrane. Fistula test induces a nystagmus and she has gross imbalance on Romberg's test. What is the most likely diagnosis?

A Lateral semicircular canal fistula

B Superior semicircular canal fistula

C Perilymphatic fistula

D Posterior semicircular canal fistula

E Tegmen dehiscence

51. A 24-year-old male presents to the emergency department with a 36-hour history of significant persistent vertigo. He has no ear pain or discharge, but has noticed left-sided tinnitus and hearing loss. He has no headache and no visual auras. He has had no prior episodes. On examination his tympanic membranes are unremarkable. He has nystagmus to the left side and his tuning forks suggest a left-sided sensorineural hearing loss. What is the most likely diagnosis?

A Labyrinthitis

B Vestibular migraine

C Vestibular neuronitis

D Stroke

E Meniere's disease

52. A 48-year-old man presents with a history of acute vertigo that started this morning and you suspect acute left vestibular failure. On examination there is a horizontal-rotational nystagmus that increases when the patient gazes towards the right side. What phenomenon is consistent with these findings?

A Romberg's test

B Hering's law

C Alexander's law

D Ewald's second law

E Herrington's law

53. A 35-year-old male presents to the clinic with 4 years of spontaneous episodes of imbalance and some drop-attacks. He describes each one as slightly different, but generally describes the room spinning

for several hours associated with sickness. He is getting episodes on a weekly basis. It is having a significant effect on his life, and he is scared to leave the house. His ear examination is normal and he has general imbalance on Romberg's test. His audiogram shows a profound sensorineural hearing loss on the right with normal hearing on the left. He has cut out salt from his diet and been commenced on betahistine and bendroflumethiazide for the last 2 years. He has also had several courses of intratympanic steroid injections to his right ear. He is keen for a definitive solution to his problem. What is the most reasonable definitive step in management in this case?

A Right labyrinthectomy

B Right endolymphatic sac decompression and duct ligation

C Right vestibular neurectomy

D Right intratympanic gentamicin injection

E Right myringotomy and grommet

54. A 66-year-old female has been experiencing episodes of vertigo lasting less than a minute whenever she turns in bed. This all started following a fall 3 months ago. She has a normal ear examination and audiogram. She has a positive Dix-Hallpike test to the left. Which of the following best describes the manoeuvre to treat this condition?

A Turn the patient's head to the right for 1 minute, then towards the floor on the right side, then sit the patient up on the right side of the bed

B Turn the patient's head to the left for 1 minute, then towards the floor on the left side, then sit the patient up on the left side of the bed

C Turn the patient's head to the right side for 1 minute, then to the left side, then to the right side again, then sit the patient up on the right side of the bed

D Turn the patient's head to the left side for 1 minute, then to the right side, then to the left side again, then sit the patient up on the left side of the bed

E Turn the patient's head to the left side for 5 minutes, then sit them up

55. **A 36-year-old female has had trouble-some symptoms of left-sided autophony, brain-fog and imbalance on loud noises, and is able to hear her eyeballs moving. Her high-resolution CT scan shows a defect of the inner ear on the left side. Which of the following results is most useful to help confirm her diagnosis?**
    A Cervical Vestibular evoked myogenic potential (VEMP): lower threshold and higher amplitude on left
    B Cervical VEMP: lower threshold and higher amplitude on right
    C Left supranormal bone conduction
    D Left-sided conductive hearing loss
    E Right supranormal bone conduction

56. **A 36-year-old female has had trouble-some symptoms of autophony, brain-fog, imbalance with loud-noises and an ability to hear her eyeballs moving. Her high-resolution CT scan shows a defect of the inner ear on the left side. Which of the following features is most likely to be present during her clinical examination?**
    A Positive fistula test on the right
    B Weber to the right
    C Tuning fork heard in left ear when placed on elbow
    D Dix-Hallpike positive on left
    E Rinne negative on right

57. **A 64-year-old woman has had multiple tympanomastoid operations for cholesteatoma with unsuccessful ossiculoplasties but preserved bone conduction thresholds. Conventional hearing aids precipitate a discharging ear and she is being considered for middle ear implantation. Which of the following would be a negative indicator for active middle ear implantation?**
    A Absent stapes
    B False fundus
    C. Progressive hearing loss

D. Recurrent otitis externa

E Stable air conduction thresholds of 60 dB from 0.5–4 kHz

58. **A 35-year-old male is involved in a road traffic accident and is noted to have a temporal bone fracture on acute imaging. He presents to your outpatient clinic 4 months later with reduced hearing. An audiogram demonstrated a maximal conductive hearing loss with an air-bone gap of 60 dB on the affected side. A CT scan of the temporal bones demonstrates disruption to the ossicular chain. What is the most common type of traumatic ossicular injury seen on CT imaging?**
    A Malleus fracture
    B Incus fracture
    C Stapes fracture
    D Incudo-stapedial joint dislocation
    E Incudo-mallear joint dislocation

59. **A 35-year-old male is involved in a road traffic accident and is noted to have a temporal bone fracture on acute imaging. He presents to your outpatient clinic 4 months later with reduced hearing. An audiogram demonstrated a maximal conductive hearing loss with masked bone conduction thresholds of 20 dB on the affected side. A CT scan of the temporal bones demonstrates disruption to the ossicular chain. Which of the following statements is true?**
    A Hearing outcomes with total ossicular replacement prostheses (TORPs) are significantly better than partial ossicular replacement prostheses (PORPs)
    B Successful air-bone gap closure is considered <30 dB
    C Surgical results from ossiculoplasty prostheses remain stable over time
    D Successful air-bone gap closure is considered <20 dB
    E The status of the middle ear is not significant

60. **You are revising the mastoid cavity of a 45-year-old patient who has had previous**

canal wall down procedures for chronic mucosal otitis media. He has a shallow middle ear space and a mobile stapes footplate; you therefore decide that the best course of action is to expose the stapes footplate and graft the tympanic membrane so the middle ear consists only of the hypotypmpanum and Eustachian tube. Which type of tympanoplasty is this?

A Wullstein Type I
B Wullstein Type II
C Wullstein Type III
D Wullstein Type IV
E Wullstein Type V

61. An 8-year-old boy with known chronic mucosal otitis media has had a persistent leak of clear fluid from the ear. He then presents to A&E with purulent otorrhoea, pyrexia and a headache. A CT is obtained and the radiologist reports the presence of a Hyrtl's fissure. This fissure is a risk factor for which intracranial complication of both acute and chronic otitis media?

A Sigmoid sinus thrombosis
B Otitic hydrocephalus
C Temporal lobe abscess
D Meningitis
E Subdural abscess

62. A 6-year-old boy presents to clinic with a central, currently dry tympanic membrane perforation which has been present for 3 years. He is a keen swimmer but suffers with recurrent otorrhoea when swimming despite appropriate water precautions. The contralateral ear has a middle ear effusion. What is the most appropriate management option?

A Offer a myringoplasty
B Offer and adenoidectomy and myringoplasty
C Offer a myringoplasty and contralateral grommet
D Watch and wait with water precautions until Eustachian tube function improves
E Offer a cartilage myringoplasty

63. A 49-year-old woman attends your clinic with a history of persistent right-sided otalgia that is worse in the mornings, associated with intermittent trismus and a feeling of fullness in the ear. Clinical and audiological examination of the ear are entirely normal. You suspect that this is a temporomandibular joint dysfunction. Which is the most reliable diagnostic clinical finding in TMJ dysfunction?

A MRI changes
B Trismus
C Joint crepitus
D Normal ear examination
E Tenderness of the masticatory muscles

64. A patient attends clinic with a perforated tympanic membrane from which they have had a chronic, malodorous discharge. On examination they have a wet perforation with mucoid discharge with visible inflamed middle ear mucosa. Which organism is most commonly involved in chronic suppurative otitis media?

A *Haemophilus influenzae*
B *Bacteroides fragilis*
C *Moraxella catarrhalis*
D *Pseudomonas aeruginosa*
E *Staphylococcus aureus*

65. A 45-year-old man presents with complaints of difficulty understanding speech, especially in noisy environments. Neurological examination is normal. Pure tone audiometry shows hearing thresholds within normal limits. Stapedial reflex thresholds are absent. Otoacoustic emissions (OAEs) are normal. Acoustic brainstem responses (ABR) are absent. Which of the following is most likely the cause of his symptoms?

A Abnormal outer hair cell function
B Abnormal neural synchrony
C Language developmental disorder
D Abnormal middle ear function
E ADHD

66. A patient attends otology clinic with a conductive hearing loss. On examination their right tympanic membrane is adherent to the cochlear promontory and does not lift on Valsalva. This retraction would be described as:
    A Tos II
    B Tos III
    C Tos IV
    D Sadé III
    E Sadé IV

67. A child visits the microtia clinic and is found to have a conductive hearing loss. Genetic testing confirms an autosomal dominant frameshift mutation in the *TCOF1* gene, and the child is diagnosed with Treacher Collins syndrome. All the following phenotypes are commonly associated with this syndrome *except*:
    A Coloboma
    B Slanting palpebral fissures
    C Mandibular hypoplasia/micrognathia
    D Intellectual disability
    E Tracheostomy requirement

68. A previously healthy 60-year-old individual arrives at the emergency department, complaining of intense throbbing pain concentrated around the temple region, along with hearing impairment that has developed within the past 36 hours. The attending nurse informs you that the patient has already been administered oral opiate medication to help with the pain. Upon otoscopy examination, the patient experiences significant tenderness. The otoscopy shows an erythematous external auditory meatus with stenosis, but the visualised section of tympanic membrane appears normal. The patient's vision remains unaffected. Based on this clinical presentation, what is the most probable diagnosis?
    A Temporal arteritis
    B Contact dermatitis

C First branchial cleft anomaly
D Otitis externa
E Furuncle

69. A 68-year-old woman presents to your clinic with a history of acute dizziness that started 4 weeks ago following an upper respiratory tract infection. She had severe continuous dizziness for 3 days that affected her ability to walk. This was associated with nausea and vomiting but no hearing loss or tinnitus. She still feels unsteady when walking especially in the dark. Later, she developed recurrent episodes of brief dizziness that are triggered by head movements. What is the most likely initial diagnosis?
    A Benign paroxysmal positional vertigo (BPPV)
    B Endolymphatic hydrops
    C Vestibular neuronitis
    D Acute labyrinthitis
    E Multiple sclerosis

70. A 43-year-old woman presents with a sudden onset of severe vertigo and left hearing loss started yesterday. Neurological exam was normal. Dix-Hallpike manoeuvre is negative. Which nystagmus would you expect to see in this case?
    A Bidirectional nystagmus that is enhanced by removal of optic fixation
    B Vertical nystagmus that is unaffected by optic fixation
    C Unidirectional horizontal-torsional nystagmus to the right that is enhanced by removal of optic fixation
    D Unidirectional horizontal-torsional nystagmus to the left that is diminished by removal of optic fixation
    E Unidirectional horizontal-torsional nystagmus to the left that is enhanced by removal of optic fixation

71. A patient presents to clinic with unilateral otalgia, pruritis and otorrhoea for several

months. On examination, there is minimal inflammation of the external ear canal with no black conidiophores or white filamentous hyphae. The tympanic membrane appears reddened and swollen but there is no perforation. Audiometric thresholds show a mild conductive hearing loss and a type A tympanogram. The most likely diagnosis is:

A Bullous myringitis
B Granular myringitis
C Otomycosis
D Otitis externa
E Tympanosclerosis

72. An elderly non-diabetic patient is referred to your outpatient clinic with a chronic dull otalgia, hearing loss and otorrhoea with normal facial nerve function for several months. On examination there is excessive cerumen without granulations in the external auditory canal; following microsuction, a large keratin plug was removed revealing an area of osteonecrosis with sequestration lacking epithelium. The tympanic membrane is normal and the facial nerve is intact. What is the optimal treatment?

A Canalplasty
B IV and topical antibiotics
C Lateral temporal bone resection and adjuvant radiotherapy
D Canal wall down surgery followed by reconstruction of canal wall
E Life-long microsuction

73. A 70-year-old man with type II diabetes mellitus attends a follow up outpatients clinic appointment for repeat microsuction of his otitis externa. Since his last attendance one week ago, he has developed an ipsilateral House-Brackmann grade IV facial palsy and is having difficulty sleeping due to severe otalgia. On examination you notice granulation tissue at the bony-cartilaginous junction. Which of the following is true in relation to this condition?

A A CT scan of the temporal bones will likely reveal a malignant neoplasm infiltrating the left skull base
B The most likely causative microbe is Aspergillus
C *Staphylococcus aureus* and MRSA are more prevalent in non-diabetic patients
D Surgical debridement improves long-term outcomes of facial palsy recovery
E Single-agent antimicrobial treatment is unsuitable to treat the pathology

74. A 44-year-old keen open water swimmer attends the outpatient clinic because they frequently experience ear infections. On examination of both ears, there are multiple hard projections within the external auditory canal of varying sizes partially obscuring normal tympanic membranes. What would be the expected histological results for these lesions?

A Lamellar bone formation with parallel, concentric layers of subperiosteal bone with abundant osteocytes
B Mass of cancellous bone composed of trabeculae of bone and fibrofatty marrow
C Keratinising stratified squamous epithelium with squamous debris and evidence of bone sequestration
D Chronic inflammation within the subepithelial tissues with evidence of epithelial hyperplasia
E Poorly differentiated squamous epithelium with perineural invasion and a high mitotic count

75. A 36-year-old woman was referred from her GP for evaluation of her recurrent episodes of dizziness that are associated with headaches. Each episode lasts for several hours and impairs her ability to carry on her daily activities. The episodes are occasionally preceded by, or associated with, visual disturbances and phonophobia. Between episodes she is entirely asymptomatic. Her symptoms persist despite over-the-counter remedies.

She also describes a history of motion sickness. Vestibular and neurological examination including examination of the cranial nerves was entirely unremarkable. Otoscopy was unremarkable as well. Pure tone audiometry was normal. Based on her clinical presentation, which of the following investigations is most useful to help confirm the diagnosis?

A MRI brain
B Electro/videonystagmography
C Ocular vestibular evoked myogenic potentials (VEMPs)
D Video head impulse testing (HIT)
E CT head

76. You conduct Rinne tuning fork tests on a pre-operative patient due to undergo a tympanoplasty. Using a 256 Hz fork, bone conduction is perceived louder than air conduction but when using the 512 Hz fork air conduction is perceived louder. What is the likely air-bone gap on the patient's audiogram?

A ≤15 dB
B 15–25 dB
C 25–35 dB
D 35–45 dB
E ≥45 dB

77. A 35-year-old fit and well male returns to the otology outpatients for a routine follow-up appointment. He has experienced multiple ear infections in his left ear and has a mild conductive hearing loss with a 5–15 dB air-bone gap. The hearing in his right ear is normal. He has not had any previous surgery on either of his ears. A colleague has previously documented that he has a Sadé grade 3 retraction. Which of the following would you expect to see on microscopy examination?

A Atelectatic tympanic membrane with perforation
B Retraction onto the incus
C Adhesion onto the promontory
D Slight retraction of the pars tensa
E Retraction onto the promontory, but not adherent

78. You are performing a translabyrinthine approach to the cerebellopontine angle (CPA). You have successfully skeletonised the middle and posterior fossa dura and the sigmoid sinus and identified the jugular bulb. The next stroke of your drill opens the cochlear aqueduct and there is CSF egress. Your trainer now instructs you to NOT drill further inferiorly to avoid damage to which structure?

A Cochlea
B Petrous carotid artery
C Internal auditory meatus
D Lower cranial nerves
E Vestibule

79. A 21-year-old male presents with right-sided hearing loss and tinnitus. Non-contrast MRI of the internal auditory meatus shows a 3 cm right cerebellopontine angle lesion and a left-sided lesion completely within the internal auditory canal. He has no other neuro-otological symptoms. What is the most appropriate next step in his management?

A Rescan in 6 months to assess for growth
B Post-contrast MRI IAM
C Post-contrast MRI whole brain and spine
D Refer to clinical genetics
E Refer for consideration of Avastin treatment

80. A 50-year-old man is brought in by ambulance to the emergency department at midnight after being found on the floor at home confused and unable to mobilise. His family report a 5-year history of left-sided hearing loss and more recently worsening balance and left facial numbness. Facial movement is normal. CT scanning shows hydrocephalus with a large left cerebellopontine angle (CPA) mass. MRI scanning confirms a 5 cm vestibular schwannoma causing compression of the brainstem.

**What is the most appropriate next defini-
tive step in management?**

A Lumbar puncture in the emergency
department

B Emergency theatre tonight for VP
shunt insertion

C Emergency theatre tonight for
tumour resection via translabyrinthine
approach

D Next available elective list for VP shunt
insertion and tumour resection via
middle cranial fossa approach

E Next available elective list for VP shunt
insertion and tumour resection via
retrosigmoid approach

81. **An 80-year-old patient presents with
left-sided hearing loss. She has a history of breast cancer treated with
radical mastectomy and adjuvant
radiotherapy 35 years ago. She is
otherwise fit and well. The radiology
registrar calls you and describes a
cerebellopontine angle lesion involving the internal auditory meatus which
enhances on post-contrast MRI and has
flecks of calcification. CT shows hyperostosis of the adjacent bone. What is
the most likely pathology in view of the
radiology findings described?**

A Vestibular schwannoma

B Meningioma

C Facial nerve schwannoma

D Ependymoma

E Metastasis from breast cancer

82. **What is the clinical importance of the
bony vertical crest (Bill's bar) during dissection of the internal auditory
meatus (IAM)?**

A Divides the facial nerve from the
cochlear nerve

B Divides the facial nerve from the
superior vestibular nerve

C Divides the superior from the inferior
vestibular nerve

D Divides the inferior vestibular from the
cochlear nerve

E Divides the facial nerve from the nervus intermedius

83. **A 29-year-old female patient presents
to the emergency department with a
painful right ear and ipsilateral House-
Brackmann grade 4 facial weakness which started 3 days ago. She
is started on a course of oral steroids
and antivirals. She works as a model.
She asks if any investigations are
available to assess the likelihood of
recovery of her facial function. Which
of the following investigations would
be the most appropriate at this point
in time to predict her facial nerve
recovery?**

A Stapedial (acoustic) reflex testing

B PTA and tympanometry

C Electroneuronography (ENoG)

D Electromyography (EMG)

E MRI scan

84. **A 21-year-old female patient has a
known left facial schwannoma centred
at the geniculate ganglion. She has
no known genetic tumour predisposition. She presents to your clinic with a
deterioration in left-sided facial function from House-Brackmann grade 1
to 2. Her hearing is normal. Scanning
shows a 2 mm increase in size over the
past 12 months. What is the best option
to preserve her facial function?**

A Resection of the tumour via middle
fossa approach with end-to-end
anastomosis

B Resection of the tumour via trans-
mastoid approach with facial-
hypoglossal anastomosis

C Stereotactic radiosurgery

D Decompression of the facial nerve via
middle fossa approach

E Decompression of the facial nerve via
the trans-mastoid approach

85. **A 65-year-old patient is day 3 post-op
translabyrinthine resection of a 4 cm right
vestibular schwannoma. His bandage
was removed at day 2 and the nursing
staff report an ongoing leak of clear fluid
from the inferior part of the post-auricular
wound through a gap in the skin sutures.**

His neurological examination is normal, he has been afebrile since surgery, and bloodwork shows a down-trending CRP. What would be the next most appropriate step in the management of this patient?

A Suture to leakage site

B Lumbar puncture

C CT head

D Lumbar drain

E Return to theatre for repacking of the Eustachian tube and blind sac closure of the ear canal

86. A 24-year-old male patient presents with intermittent bleeding from his left ear on a background of several years of decreased ipsilateral hearing. On examination there is a red mass filling the ear canal which bleeds profusely on instrumentation. You organise a post-contrast CT and MRI scan which shows an enhancing mass in the middle ear extending into the temporal bone. The remainder of his cranial nerve examination is normal. What are the next most appropriate steps in the management of this patient?

A Biopsy for histology, MDT discussion, referral to clinical genetics

B Plasma metanephrines, embolisation of lesion, then trans-mastoid resection

C FBC, plasma metanephrines, referral to clinical genetics

D DOTATATE PET-CT, plasma metanephrines, referral to clinical genetics

E MRI abdomen and pelvis, plasma metanephrines, referral to clinical genetics

87. A 12-month-old patient with bilateral profound sensorineural hearing loss is being assessed for cochlear implantation. As part of the work-up an inner ear deformity is suspected on MRI scanning and confirmed on CT scanning. The MDT decision is that cochlear implantation is not possible. Which of these inner ear deformities is most likely to have been identified?

A Common cavity

B Wide vestibular aqueduct

C Michel deformity

D Mondini malformation

E Incomplete partition of the cochlea

88. A 15-year-old boy is undergoing cochlear implant assessment for progressive hearing loss. Audiogram confirms he has a bilateral normal to profound sensorineural hearing loss, with profound loss in all thresholds tested beyond 1 kHz. On questioning his parents, it emerges that he is somewhat clumsy and has been bumping into things and falling over and has hit his head on occasion. What is the next best definitive test to specifically investigate the aetiology of the hearing loss in this patient?

A Tympanogram

B Vestibular function testing

C CT temporal bones

D Thyroid function test

E Stapedial reflexes

89. A 15-year-old boy is being seen in clinic for evaluation of cochlear implantation. His radiological investigations reveal normal anatomy on MRI and CT, and he has been deemed a candidate for cochlear implantation. His parents are worried about loss of his low frequency hearing post procedure. Which of the following surgical factors are associated with best likelihood of residual hearing preservation in cochlear implantation? Choose the best option from the following choices:

A Slow insertion of electrode

B Perioperative parenteral steroids

C Perioperative antibiotics

D Ensuring no blood enters upon opening of round window membrane

E A, B and D

90. A 70-year-old patient underwent cochlear implantation 12 days ago. The procedure was straightforward, with correct and full insertion confirmed with X-ray intra-operatively. She has a post-operative cone-beam CT

scan, per the protocol of the unit, prior to switch-on. It is then noticed that 3 electrodes appear to be lying outside the cochlea. What is the next best course of action?

A Obtain electrocochleography (ECoG)
B Obtain baseline pure tone audiogram (PTA), unaided
C Immediate device integrity check
D Plan for return to theatre, with re-insertion of the implant
E Proceed as normal to audiological switch-on in 6–8 weeks

91. An 11-year-old boy recently repatriated from India has arrived to the paediatric intensive care unit intubated and ventilated. He has an acute history of fever, ear pain and seizures. His condition has been made stable; however, inflammatory markers remain persistently raised. Examination of the affected ear reveals mild post-aural fullness but no fluctuance on palpation, and an erythematous tympanic membrane. MRI and CT head with contrast confirm the presence of a very small intracranial abscess, as well as a small subperiosteal mastoid collection. The neurosurgical team propose to manage the intracranial collection medically, and have contacted you for urgent opinion. Choose the best definitive treatment from the list:

A Broad spectrum IV antibiotics with CNS penetration
B Commence anti-seizure medications following urgent neurology consultation
C Cortical mastoidectomy and grommet insertion on emergency list
D Incision and drainage of post-aural collection on emergency list
E Myringotomy and grommet insertion on emergency list

92. A 40-year-old female presents with a long-standing history of right-sided hearing loss. She has dysmorphic features more marked on the right,

along with microtia. There is no evident external auditory canal, only a small remnant of cartilage superiorly and evidence of a small lobule. CT temporal bones is undertaken revealing a normal middle ear space, normal round and oval windows, a present stapes superstructure and a normal malleus and facial nerve but malformed incus with unclear articulation with stapes. Choose the single best option reflecting her Jahrsdoerfer grading:

A 12
B 4
C 6
D 8
E 5

93. A 20-year-old sustains significant head injuries following a road traffic collision. ATLS protocol is followed. He is intubated, ventilated, stabilised and admitted to ITU. He is noted to have blood-stained discharge from the left ear, which is intermittently clear. Bedside examination is difficult with evidence of clotted blood, mixed with clear serous discharge and post-aural ecchymoses. A CT scan is undertaken the same day, revealing an otic capsule-involving temporal bone fracture, with possible involvement of perigeniculate facial nerve. Choose the next best management option:

A Commence broad spectrum IV antibiotics
B Serial ENoG testing
C EMG testing
D Auditory brainstem response (ABR)
E Send sample of fluid from ear for beta 2 transferrin

94. A 30-year-old notices tinnitus and reduced hearing following an electronic music concert. She has no prior otological history and denies any recreational drug use. She attends clinic one week later, concerned due to her

severe persistent tinnitus and ongoing reduced hearing. She has no vertigo. Select the single most accurate statement describing this scenario:

A Damage to inner ear cells results in noise-induced hearing loss

B This patient will not sustain permanent hearing loss due to the presence of stapedial reflex

C She is likely to be experiencing a temporary threshold shift

D She is likely to be experiencing a permanent threshold shift

E The sustained exposure to noise is less likely to result in lasting damage

95. A retired saxophonist who is an amateur chorister at the local church has started to note worsening symptoms of vertigo and sensitivity to sound when the organ is playing while he is standing in close proximity. In addition, he has started to find his own voice extremely loud when singing. This is accompanied by a sensation of aural fullness, tinnitus and what he calls "brain fog". He uses hearing aids bilaterally. He reports that his mother underwent stapes surgery recently. Select the most likely diagnosis:

A Otosclerosis

B Patulous Eustachian tube

C Superior semicircular canal dehiscence syndrome

D Hyperacusis

E Meniere's disease

96. A patient attends your clinic with daily autophony, vertigo induced by loud noises, tinnitus and a perceived a deterioration in hearing. His symptoms have now curtailed his ability to sing in choir, with significant impact on his quality of life. He wishes to discuss interventions. Select the next best investigation to confirm diagnosis:

A Pure tone audiometry

B Stapedial reflexes

C Cervical VEMPs

D CT head

E Tympanometry

97. A 40-year-old woman presents to your clinic with recurrent episodes of dizziness, associated with nausea, vomiting and some unsteadiness. The dizziness is frequently associated with headache. Her episodes are frequent and last from 5 minutes to 48 hours. Which of the following features would be most suggestive of her diagnosis?

A Dizziness that is triggered by loud noise

B Dizziness that is triggered by prolonged standing

C Dizziness that is triggered by moving in bed or abrupt head movements

D Dizziness that is triggered by stress or anxiety

E Dizziness that is triggered in the dark

98. A 47-year-old lady is seen for recurrent episodes of dizziness and headache that are associated with some dietary triggers. Specific investigations may reveal:

A Reduced threshold on cervical VEMP

B Increased time constants seen on rotational testing

C Loss of normal fluid signal in the inner ear on MRI IAM

D Sustained low frequency hearing loss on pure tone audiometry

E Absent threshold on cervical VEMP

99. A 47-year-old man is being evaluated for acute dizziness associated with nausea, vomiting and significant imbalance that started 3 days ago. Which of the following tests is best used to evaluate his saccular function:

A Bithermal caloric testing

B Cervical VEMPs

C Ocular VEMPs

D Subjective visual vertical

E Video HIT

ANSWERS

Otology

1. Answer C

In this scenario, ossiculoplasty is not feasible since blind sac closure surgery will have left the patient without a functional ear canal and tympanic membrane. For this reason, an air conduction hearing aid is likely to be audiologically ineffective and difficult to wear. The patient's bone conduction threshold of 50 dB in the affected ear means he would be beyond the threshold for a Bonebridge implant to provide restoration of binaural stimulation. Audiometrically he is in criteria for both an OSIA implant and a percutaneous bone conduction implant. However, the recent cholesteatoma clearance is likely to require diffusion weighted MRI (dwMRI) surveillance in the first five years to detect recurrence. The presence of an OSIA would cause a shadow over the field on an MRI scan, meaning the only way to detect recurrence would be with elective revision surgery. Therefore, percutaneous bone-anchored hearing implant (which has minimal MRI shadow) is the most appropriate answer since the question states that the patient wants help imminently. The alternative options of a softband bone conduction aid or active middle ear implant would also be acceptable choices but are not given as options.

2. Answer E

Palatal myoclonus features rhythmic involuntary movements of the soft palate and pharynx. This causes the tensor veli palatini and levator veli palatini muscles to pull on the Eustachian tube. The resulting sound is transmitted directly to the middle ear. This is therefore a non-vascular cause of pulsatile tinnitus and hence is not synchronous with the heart rate. It usually produces a clicking sound, which may be objective i.e. heard by others. Palatal myoclonus may be related to brainstem pathology (pathology in the triangle of Guillain-Mollaret/dentato-rubro-olivary pathway), for which an MRI scan is important in the diagnosis but more commonly it is idiopathic. Diagnosis is made by observing palatal spasms by direct examination or nasendoscopy. Treatment includes muscle relaxants or EMG-guided Botox injections.

3. Answer D

Sound localisation relies on the brain's assimilation of differences in volume and timing between left and right aural input. In unilateral profound hearing loss, both a CROS aid and bone conduction devices reduce the head shadow effect by routing all sound through the contralateral vestibulocochlear nerve. Therefore, in such cases, binaural information is not restored and therefore effects on localisation are limited at best. If hearing in the affected ear were in aidable territory, then this would be the most important factor in the ability to restore binaural hearing. Since the question states a profound hearing loss in the affected ear, one would not expect to benefit from a conventional acoustic hearing aid. Ipsilateral cochlear implantation, whilst not currently funded in the UK NHS for single-sided deafness, would aim to restore access to inter-aural information. Both duration of deafness and status of the ipsilateral vestibulocochlear nerve are important prognostic factors in cochlear implantation, but a shorter (and hence more favourable) duration of deafness may not be enough to overcome a poorly functioning vestibulocochlear nerve, hence the latter is the most appropriate answer.

4. **Answer C**

The tensor tympani arises from the Eustachian tube, petrous temporal bone and the greater wing of the sphenoid. It passes into the protympanic space covered by the semicanal for the tensor tympani. The point at which the tensor tympani gives off a tendon inserting into the malleus neck is called the processus cochleariformis. This is a reliable landmark in tympanomastoid surgery since it is relatively resistant to erosion. Cochleariform means 'spoon-shaped' rather than being related to the cochlea. The geniculate ganglion, located at the first genu of the facial nerve, is immediately superior to this bony process. It lies in a bony tunnel and in a more medial plane. The ganglion contains cell bodies of the fibres responsible for carrying taste sensation from the anterior two thirds of the tongue. Additionally, the ganglion contributes to the sensory innovation of areas such as the palate, concha and ear canal. From the geniculate ganglion the facial nerve passes in the fallopian canal, which can be found to be dehiscent, superior to the stapes and oval window, and inferior to the lateral semicircular canal towards its second genu. The supratubal recess lies anteriorly and inferiorly relative to the processus cochleariformis. The cog and malleus head lie in a more lateral and superior position.

5. **Answer A**

Infected osteoradionecrosis and necrotising otitis externa may present very similarly. Non-resolving otitis externa with night pain, ear canal granulations and intractable pain should alert the clinician. High-resolution CT scanning reveals bony erosion and demineralisation characteristic of both conditions. The history distinguishes the two, with a history of local radiotherapy making osteoradionecrosis the most likely diagnosis. A history of diabetes and other diseases of immunocompromise may point more towards necrotising otitis externa. *Pseudomonas aeruginosa* may be grown in both conditions. In necrotising otitis externa, non-echo planar diffusion-weighted MRI (non-EPI DWI) has been shown to be valuable in assessing disease extent and treatment response over conventional T1 and T2 weighted sequences. Technetium-99m methylene diphosphonate (Tc99m MDP) scanning has been used as a sensitive tool for detecting bony changes but is non-specific and cannot be relied on to differentiate active infection from resolution and new bone formation. Tagged white blood cell scans, e.g. Gallium 67, have utility in monitoring treatment response. Recently positron emission tomography-MRI (PET-MRI) scans have been used to follow patients with skull base osteomyelitis.

6. **Answer E**

Sensation in the external auditory canal is supplied by the trigeminal, facial, glossopharyngeal and vagus nerves. Frequently, microsuction of the ear canal may stimulate patients to cough. This is caused by stimulation of the auricular branch of the vagus nerve known as Arnold's nerve. Sensory innervation of the auricle is supplied by the great auricular and lesser occipital nerves (from the C2–3 plexus) as well as Arnold's nerve, the auriculotemporal nerve (branch of the mandibular branch of the trigeminal) and the facial nerve. There is not typically glossopharyngeal afferent supply to the auricle. The tympanic nerve (Jacobson's nerve) is a branch of the glossopharyngeal nerve that supplies sensation of the middle ear, Eustachian tube, mastoid air cells and parotid gland. Jacobson's nerve also gives parasympathetic to supply to the parotid gland via the otic ganglion and the auriculotemporal nerve.

7. **Answer C**

    The cochlea consists of three parallel canals, coiled together in a spiral around a coni-cally shaped central axis known as the modiolus. This modiolus houses the axons of central projections of the cochlear nerve which supply innervation to sensory epithelia. It also contains the blood supply to the cochlea—the cochlear artery and vein. The 'mid-dle' canal of the three parallel canals is the scala media (in between the scala tympani and scala vestibuli). The base of the scala media, the basilar membrane, contains the organ of Corti—made up of inner and outer hair cells and responsible for the tonotopic organisation of the cochlea. The stria vascularis runs along the lateral side of the scala media and is the site of endolymph production. Reissner's membrane forms the roof of the scala media, separating it from the scala vestibuli. The helicotrema is the part of the cochlea where the scala tympani and vestibuli meet. Sound energy conducted through the ossicular chain displaces incompressible perilymph along the scala vestibuli, through the helicotrema and down the scala tympani leading to 'out–in' movements of the round window. As fluid is displaced, the pressure difference across the scala media between the scala vestibuli and scala tympani moves the basilar membrane. This wave of movement stimulates the sensory cells housed in the organ of Corti.

8. **Answer A**

    The three key auditory factors in sound localisation are processing of inter-aural timing dif-ference, processing of inter-aural volume difference, and cues provided by pinna shape. The pinna comprises a number of anatomical ridges and concavities. Sound waves from the horizontal and vertical planes are reflected from these structures prior to entering the ear canals, alongside waves of the original non-reflected sound. This combined sound information is then delivered via the tympanic membrane and ossicular chain to be perceived in the auditory cortex as directional and spatial representation of sound. Pinna abnormalities may therefore interfere with spatial hearing ability, even if symmetrical.

9. **Answer D**

    This stem describes a case of sudden sensorineural hearing loss presenting early. Oral corticosteroid is one of the few treatments with demonstrated efficacy and has wide-spread use. However, this patient has two concerning risk factors for systemic steroid complications—peptic ulcer disease and poorly controlled diabetes. In this case it is appropriate to opt for intratympanic steroid administration as the initial management option. Both methylprednisolone and dexamethasone are used for this purpose. The dexamethasone option here is a dose far lower than regularly used, which makes methylprednisolone the most appropriate choice.

10. **Answer C**

    In a case of delayed-onset (rather than immediate) facial palsy after tympanomas-toid surgery, one can infer that the facial nerve is structurally intact. The aetiology of delayed-onset facial weakness after surgery is often indeterminate. Reactivation of herpes simplex or varicella zoster virus is postulated as an underlying mechanism but any cause of neural inflammation or ischaemia could be responsible. Combined use of prednisone and aciclovir with or without systemic antibiotics can be considered as the first option. There is no clear difference in outcomes between early vs >7 days delayed exploration and decompression in cases of delayed complete palsy. It is appropriate to involve a more experienced colleague or refer to a regional subspecialty centre when re-exploration is required.

11. Answer D

The addition of chemotherapy provides a survival benefit in patients with non-metastatic head and neck cancer that are 70 and younger (MACH-NC meta-analysis). Cisplatin is a commonly used first-line chemotherapeutic in head and neck cancer. Unfortunately, it can cause hearing loss, necessitating a complete discussion of the risks and benefits of treatment. Proper audiological assessment is useful to guide this. If there is pre-existing hearing loss or new sensorineural hearing loss, then the patient could be switched to carboplatin which is less ototoxic despite also being a platinum-based chemotherapeutic. There have been phase 2 trials of transtympanic sodium thiosulphate but these are not given outside clinical trials. It should be noted that systemic sodium thiosulphate has recently been approved for the prevention of ototoxicity induced by cisplatin in patients over 1 month of age with non-metastatic solid tumours.

Transtympanic steroid injections are also not performed routinely, given the likely mechanism of cisplatin related hair cell death. There are concerns about systemic steroids given to prevent ototoxicity promoting the tumour lysis effect, and although steroids are routinely given for chemotherapy side effects without issue, they are generally not used for hearing loss. There is no evidence for hyperbaric oxygen in chemotherapy-related hearing loss in humans.

12. Answer D

The patient has bilateral sensorineural hearing loss and vestibulopathy secondary to the presumed aminoglycosides administration. The m.1555A→G variant (due to a single nucleotide A to G substitution) at position 1555 of the mitochondrial genome is located in the 12S ribosomal RNA gene. It is known to cause hearing loss, especially after exposure to aminoglycoside antibiotics. This can occur even at therapeutic aminoglycoside levels. This variant is inherited maternally. In this case genetic testing is important to help to counsel her children. Imaging would be useful if planning for cochlear implantation. Caloric testing assesses the vestibular ocular reflex (VOR) of the lateral canals relative to each other and therefore cannot diagnose a bilateral vestibular hypofunction. vHIT can detect covert saccades and provides canal-specific information about the VOR but is not necessary. Rotatory chair testing is able to test the lateral canal VOR and diagnose bilateral peripheral vestibulopathy; however, it is not necessary. Posturography is a functional assessment of balance and the visual, vestibular and proprioceptive inputs. In this case vestibular testing is not necessary because the diagnosis is made by the history and examination.

13. Answer B

This audiogram shows a difference of air conduction of 110 db. This immediately suggests the audiogram is not accurate. The interaural attenuation with insert headphones is 60 dB (and with over-the-ear headphones is 40 dB). This would mean that at 70 dB, the patient should hear the sound via the contralateral cochlea and should respond and the air conduction on the left would appear to be 60–70 dB. This suggests that the patient is feigning a hearing loss and refusing to acknowledge sound. The pure tone audiogram (PTA) is a subjective hearing test. Another example of a subjective test is speech recognition threshold whereby the patient is asked to repeat two-syllable 'spondee' words back. Patients can purposely choose to mishear words. The patient requires further investigation to objectively test his hearing before being offered a hearing aid. From the list, auditory brainstem response (ABR), cortical evoked response audiometry (CERA) and otoacoustic emissions (OAEs) are objective tests of hearing.

An OAE can be done quickly within minutes and tests up to the cochlear hair cells. An ABR tests up to the brainstem. CERA tests the entire auditory pathway to the cortex and is therefore the gold standard to test hearing in these cases. This test can take a significant portion of time and needs a separate appointment to be organised.

14. **Answer C**

The patient may be feigning a hearing loss. A PTA, word recognition score (WRS) and speech recognition threshold (SRT) are all subjective tests of hearing. The SRT should be consistent with the PTA and the WRS should give functional information about hearing. There are different patterns of word scores depending on the nature of the hearing loss (conductive, sensorineural or retrocochlear). Tympanometry is objective and gives information about the admittance and impedance of sound through the outer and middle ear but not the hearing. Stapedial reflexes are an objective test. In a normal ear, sound triggers a reflex at approximately 70 dB. In this case, if there is a response at both the ipsilateral and contralateral ear with both right and left stimuli, then the hearing is likely to be normal or a mild sensorineural hearing loss (SNHL). If there is no response, there may be a conductive loss or a severe SNHL. The threshold may be elevated in a moderate SNHL.

15. **Answer A**

A 13-year-old child should be able to perform a PTA without any issue. The audiogram suggests that the child was not able to allow them to accurately test his hearing. This is likely to be intentional with the history given and consistent with non-organic hearing loss rather than failure to understand and comply with the test. The motivation behind children feigning hearing loss include receiving special attention, escaping bullying and an excuse for their behaviour or academic performance. The best test to be performed at the same clinic attendance is distortion product OAE (DPOAE) because it can provide frequency-specific and ear-specific hearing thresholds. Transient Evoked OAEs present a click stimulus which is a broad range of frequencies at once. The test is not frequency-specific. Both tests are quick to perform by audiologists but the DPOAE provides frequency-specific information. Both can identify a moderate (40 dB) hearing loss or worse. There must be no conductive hearing loss in order for the test to be performed, which is confirmed by the history, normal examination and type A tympanogram. An ABR test can be completed only if the child is sleeping or lying perfectly still, relaxed and with his or her eyes closed which is why a general anaesthetic is used for non-compliant children. ABR and CERA are tests that require a separate appointment because these can take an hour or more to perform. Speech audiometry is a behavioural test that is also subject to intentional manipulation. Stapedial reflexes are tested at three frequencies and are absent in conductive hearing loss and facial nerve weakness. They can be present at mild or moderate hearing loss.

16. **Answer B**

The bilateral cookie bite hearing loss with a family history suggests genetic hearing loss. No further investigation with imaging is needed; however, genetic testing may be considered. Hearing loss prevention can be targeted to preventing noise-induced hearing loss, modifying vascular risk factors and immunisations. The Control of Noise at Work Regulations 2005 state that if noise is over 80 dB on average per day or week or a peak sound pressure over 135 dB then staff can request hearing protection. Above 85 dB on average per day or week or a peak sound pressure over 137 dB they must wear hearing protection. The daily or weekly exposure of 87 dB and peak sound pressure of 140 dB should not be exceeded. The noise in a nightclub can be around 100 dB. Managing vascular risk factors is important to prevent deterioration of cochlear function due to vascular compromise. Furosemide only induces temporary hearing loss, but rarely permanent deafness can occur in severe acute or chronic renal failure or with other ototoxic drugs. There is no role for prednisolone in chronic gradual hearing loss.

17. Answer E

This patient has a congenital aural atresia which is the absence of a patent ear canal. This can occur with or without microtia. This occurs due to the failure of invagination of the ear canal which can also result in an abnormal ear drum. Most often, this disruption occurs randomly, but it is related to several syndromes, including Goldenhaar, Treacher Collins and Crouzon syndromes. Cosmetic pinna reconstruction surgery is usually performed toward the end of the first decade of life, when substantial mastoid development has occurred. Hearing improvement after atresia repair is modest (approximately 25 dB) but may be sufficient to allow use of a conventional hearing aid. One of the major risks of this surgery is injury to the facial nerve or the dura of the middle cranial fossa. As such, its use in the UK is very limited if performed at all. A middle ear implant has the potential benefit of offering side-specific information with subsequent benefit to sound localisation which is likely to be important to an amateur footballer. In this case a stapes coupler is likely to be the most reliable location of transducer attachment, since formation of the malleus and incus occurs at the same time as invagination of the external auditory canal and therefore can also be affected (though the question does not provide CT scan information). A percutaneous bone-anchored hearing implant would also be a suitable option here and may be chosen by this patient. An active middle ear implant has the potential benefits of purely ipsilateral cochlear stimulation and greater sound authenticity, though the patient should be counselled regarding comparatively greater surgical risks. Transcutaneous implantable bone conduction devices are potential options here, though are not listed as options. A conventional hearing aid is not suitable since there is no passage for air conduction. A CROS aid will not stimulate the cochlea on the affected side.

18. Answer D

The main complications of a percutaneous BAHA are skin complications. These complications have reduced because the surgical technique now requires less soft tissue dissection. The patient says she cannot use her BAHA and needs it for work. She can use the processor she already has and attach it to a softband as a temporary measure which would be the quickest option for her. She then could choose between revising the skin issue to salvage the BAHA, having a new BAHA at a different site or choosing an implantable device depending on her audiogram. In terms of surgical waiting list time, either revising her BAHA or inserting a new one could be done under a local anaesthetic and performed with a shorter waiting time.

19. Answer B

The patient has a retrocochlear cause of hearing loss and these patients often have a significantly lower word recognition score than one would expect from their audiogram. The word recognition score can use monosyllabic words or spondees presented to the patients and the amplification is increased until a plateau is reached. In conductive hearing loss, increased amplification should allow for a 100% score. In SNHL, increased amplification does not reach 100%. In patients a low score despite amplification suggests that a hearing aid which works by amplification may not be sat-isfactory for the patient. In a retrocochlear cause, there is rollover in which amplification reduces the ability to correctly hear the phonemes and shows that a hearing aid on that side is unlikely to be useful. In this case the options would then be a bone conduc-tion hearing device or contralateral routing of sound (CROS) aid. Good word recogni-tion scores predict favourable response to amplification, since they indicate that the patient can understand words if they are amplified to comfortable levels.

20. **Answer A**

    This patient has a severe hearing loss so in-the-canal (ITC), completely-in-canal (CIC) and invisible-in-canal (IIC) aids are unlikely to be able to provide her enough amplifi-cation. The CIC and IIC aids require the ear canal to be wide enough to be inserted. They often require a specialist to insert them and have small batteries which frequently need to be replaced. With this patient's arthritis, the easiest hearing aid to use is a behind-the-ear aid. An open-designed ear dome prevents the occlusion effect but also increases likelihood of acoustic feedback between the dome and the micro-phone. Therefore, such use is limited in mild to moderate hearing loss. She could have a behind-the-ear aid with a custom mould with a vent to reduce the occlusion effect. A receiver-in-the-ear aid has the microphone in the tip and is useful to overcome acoustic feedback by increasing the distance between the microphone and speaker. The behind-the-ear component is therefore smaller and cosmetically more favourable but it can require fine dexterity to insert. The in-the-ear aid can only be seen from the side and the in-the-canal aid is even less visible. Both require fine dexterity to insert and have small batteries and issues with feedback. Body-worn hearing aids are rarely worn now since the power of conventional hearing aids has matched them. Only the BTE or, very occasionally, the RITE type is available via NHS care in the UK. The main auditory difficulties encountered in hearing aid use are inadequate amplification, occlusion and feedback. Other side effects include recurrent otitis externa, wax build-up, skin irritation from an uncomfortable mould or a contact dermatitis.

21. **Answer E**

    With increasing age, there is loss of inner and outer hair cells within the cochlea as well as loss of spiral ganglion cells and central auditory neurons. This typically results in a high-frequency sensorineural hearing loss that progresses slowly over time. Older patients with presbycusis therefore may also have more diminished speech discrimina-tion than younger patients with the same level of pure-tone averages.

    For a given pure-tone hearing loss, the speech discrimination decreases with aging. Schuknecht described four patterns of presbycusis. In sensory presbycusis there is loss of hair cells which results in an abruptly sloping pattern and excellent speech discrimi-nation. In neural presbycusis there is loss of cochlear neurons resulting in a variably downsloping audiogram and poor speech discrimination. In strial presbycusis the stria vascularis is affected and there is a flat pure-tone audiogram with excellent speech discrimination. Conductive presbycusis is a theoretical category of presbycusis which affects the basilar membrane resulting in a gradually sloping high-frequency and poor speech discrimination.

    The presented scenario likely describes neural presbycusis. Loudness recruitment is a phenomenon in sensorineural hearing loss whereby sounds are perceived to become rapidly louder with increasing sound levels. This means that the dynamic range of hearing is reduced. This leads to the affected person requesting for people to speak louder, and then to complain that that person is shouting when they speak a little louder. The cocktail party effect is the ability of the higher auditory pathway to focus their listening to a particular stimulus. Patients with sensorineural hearing loss may complain of speech-in-noise processing. Modern hearing aids attempt to combat this with directional microphones and software but will always to some degree amplify both speech and noise. Paracusis of Willis is a phenomenon in which people with a conductive hearing loss, especially otosclerosis, are able to hear speech better in noisy environments. This is thought to be due to the fact that speakers will raise their voices to combat the noisy environment and amplification is able to achieve 100% word recognition in conductive hearing loss.

22. Answer B

This patient has a contact dermatitis to the hearing aids rather than otitis externa. This can be to a variety of materials including the silicone, plastic casing or paint. Patients can be referred to dermatology to have patch testing to confirm an allergy. Audiologists are able to tackle this by changing the hearing aid. If recurrent otitis externa secondary to the hearing aid is an issue, the audiologist may be able to tackle this with creation of ventilation holes. If irritation was suspected due to the shape of the mould, they could adjust this. In the absence of an otitis externa, drops would not be useful. Steroid ointment is a temporary solution and should be avoided long term.

23. Answer D

The incidence of sensorineural hearing loss in children with bacterial meningitis has been reported at 10% and is usually profound and irreversible. The pathway is due to infection traveling from the subarachnoid space via the CSF to the cochlear aqueduct and then the organ of Corti. As a consequence of endosteal inflammation, new bone may be laid down within the cochlear lumen and cause partial or total obliteration of the lumen (osteoneogenesis resulting in cochlear ossificans). There is also disruption of the auditory processing pathway in the central nervous system and the audiologic outcomes are difficult to predict, especially in the presence of cochlear ossification. Ossification can occur 3 weeks after the onset of meningitis and so prompt referral is essential. Clinicians should order imaging to prevent delays simultaneously. Only an MRI is necessary in a child to prevent radiation exposure. In an adult a CT with or without MRI is useful. Giving steroids orally or transtympanically is unlikely to reverse the hearing loss. The use of steroids to prevent cochlear ossificans is controversial. In both adults and children the recommendation would be bilateral cochlear implantation, since it is unpredictable which side will function best and there is a small window of opportunity to perform implantation.

24. Answer C

The aim of the NHS newborn hearing screening programme in England (NHSP) is the identification of permanent childhood hearing impairment (PCHI) in newborn babies which is defined as a bilateral permanent hearing loss averaging >= 40 dBnHL (dB normal hearing level) across 0.5 to 4 kHz. Early identification gives babies better opportunity and support to develop language, speech and communication skills. The pathways of delivery are the well baby pathway and NICU (neonatal intensive care unit) pathway. Both pathways recommend immediate audiological assessment rather than screening if there is atresia, microtia, confirmed congenital CMV (cytomegalovirus) or a programmable shunt. In the well baby pathway, the child is usually tested before discharge with AOAE. If they do not have clear responses in both ears, this is repeated at a later date. If they do not have clear responses in both ears a second time then AABR (automated ABR) is performed. If they do not have clear responses in both ears they are referred for immediate audiological assessment. If they pass their assessment but have any risk factors of syndromes associated with hearing loss (including Down's syndrome), cranio-facial abnormalities, including cleft palate/bifid uvula (and therefore subsequent risks of prolonged middle ear effusion), confirmed congenital infection (toxoplasmosis or rubella) or have been in a special care baby unit (SCBU) or NICU over 48 hours they can be referred for audiological assessment at 7 to 9 months. In the NICU pathway they are screened with both AOAE and AABR from the beginning because there is a higher risk of deafness.

25. **Answer C**

This patient has presbycusis. This has previously been described histologically as degeneration of the hair cells, neural cells, stria vascularis or basilar membrane. This age-related degeneration is contributed to by other factors such as noise trauma, vascular disease, ototoxic drugs over a lifetime. Older patients with presbycusis also have more diminished speech discrimination than younger patients with the same hearing loss on their audiogram.

The degeneration can also affect the vestibule and vestibular nerves causing imbalance. The hearing loss can also contribute to imbalance. The patient describes benefit from the hearing aids except when the speaker is farther away. As such, hearing aids may still be the preferred option over cochlear implantation, although speech discrimination testing is important in clarifying candidacy based on NICE guidance in the UK. A minister's sermon will likely sound muddled for a hearing aid wearer because a cavernous church will easily reverberate and mix speech sounds with the surrounding background noise, obscuring the words.

An FM (frequency modulation) or a DM (digital modulation) system is an assistive listening device whereby a microphone can be used to transmit sound from one area to another. This can be used by placing the device close to the speaker which will then transmit to the hearing aids. Another assistive listening device is a loop system in which a microphone connects to a wire loop which is placed around an area. This loop creates a magnetic wireless signal that is picked up by a hearing aid when it is set to the T-setting (telecoil). However, this requires the venue to be set up for this system which it may not be. He does not meet the criteria for a bone-anchored hearing aid.

26. **Answer D**

Sofradex contains acetic acid, framycetin and dexamethasone.

Ciloxan contains ciprofloxacin (3mg/ml ciprofloxacin hydrochloride without dexamethaone).

Ofloxacin is a fluoroquinolone similar to ciprofloxacin.

Gentisone HC contains gentamicin and hydrocortisone. Locorten Vioform is a combination of flumetasone (steroid) and clioquinol which is an antifungal.

27. **Answer B**

This patient has an auto-myringostapedopexy: the tympanic membrane retracts due to Eustachian tube dysfunction and has eroded the long process of the incus to be attached to the stapes head. Despite the loss of the long process, patients can often enjoy near-normal hearing due to the apposition of the tympanic membrane onto the stapes head (akin to a type 3 tympanoplasty). Such patients require serial follow-up because the retraction may develop into a cholesteatoma. Ventilation tube placement is unlikely to reverse the condition by this point. Ossiculoplasty is unlikely to yield a significantly better hearing result than the patient currently has. Tympanomastoid surgery would not be the primary option since the patient does not have a cholesteatoma, nor any recurrent infections.

Conservative management with a hearing aid assessment and serial follow-up is therefore most reasonable an option here. Indications to move to surgery would be deterioration of hearing or recurrent infections.

28. **Answer D**

    Otosclerosis is familial with a positive family history in up to 60% of cases, with studies suggesting an autosomal dominant pattern with incomplete penetrance. The process only affects the otic capsule structure and so foci do not develop on the malleus, incus or stapes superstructure since these are first and second branchial arch derivates. The process causes disorganised bony turnover and so the bone of the otic capsule is transformed from the densest bone in the body to a more histologically spongy type of bone. Otosclerosis is therefore a misnomer. When this process affects the labyrinth, this can cause sensorineural hearing loss. In addition to stapes surgery, hearing aids or no treatment are valid management options.

29. **Answer B**

    A stapes prosthesis should be sized and securely placed onto the long process of the incus. The size is determined by the distance from the vestibule to the long process of the incus with an appropriately sized prosthesis placed accordingly. An excessively long prosthesis may extend too far into the vestibule causing vertigo. In extreme cases this can also cause a sensorineural hearing loss. A prosthesis that is too short can cause fluctuating hearing loss with large movements of the tympanic membrane (such as yawning or when flying). In some cases this may also migrate out of the stapedotomy causing a further conductive hearing loss.

30. **Answer A**

    A variety of ossicular replacement prostheses can be used depending on the aspect(s) of the ossicular chain requiring reconstruction. A partial ossicular replacement prosthesis (such as a Dresden clip or a Bell prosthesis) is placed onto the stapes capitulum to bridge the gap between the tympanic membrane and the stapes in cases when the incus is absent. Where there is partial erosion of the long process of the incus, the gap between the long process and the stapes capitulum can be rebuilt with bone cement. A total ossicular replacement prosthesis is used where there is an absent stapes superstructure and so bridges between the tympanic membrane and the mobile footplate. This can be used in conjunction with a footplate prosthesis (such as a Dornhoffer shoe or omega clip) or a malleus replacement prosthesis to provide lateral stability.

31. **Answer A**

    Iatrogenic facial palsy is a rare complication of otological surgery though certain factors can make this more likely. These include instrumentation used, anatomical considerations and the use of a facial nerve monitor. Operations involving powered instruments such as drills or lasers can cause facial nerve injury through mechanical or thermal injury. Facial nerve dehiscence is a normal anatomical variant in up to 20% of the population, though this can be higher in patients with cholesteatoma in whom the disease process can cause erosion of the fallopian canal. Of the operations listed, tympanomastoid surgery for cholesteatoma therefore carries the greatest risk of iatrogenic facial palsy.

32. Answer C

Otitis media with effusion (OME) (glue ear) commonly results from poor Eustachian tube function resulting in inadequate middle ear ventilation. Craniofacial anomalies can result in dilatory Eustachian tube dysfunction. Passive cigarette smoke can cause irritation of the middle ear mucosa and subsequent goblet cell proliferation predisposing to middle ear effusion. Attending day care facilities can increase the frequency of upper respiratory tract infections which can also increase the likelihood of OME. Bottle feeding and lower socio-economic backgrounds are also associated with an increased incidence of OME.

33. Answer A

Griesinger's sign is described here which is oedema of the post-auricular soft tissues. This is secondary to thrombosis of the mastoid emissary vein secondary to acute otomastoiditis. Hitselberger's sign is hyperesthesia or anaesthesia of the posterior external auditory canal. This is sometimes seen in vestibular schwannomas due to compression of the sensory fibres of the facial nerve by the tumour. Brown's sign describes a red mass behind the tympanic membrane which blanches upon pneumatic otoscopy. This is seen in a tympanic paraganglioma. Hennebert's sign is also seen on pneumatic otoscopy and describes a positive fistula test (nystagmus and/or vertigo induced by pneumatic otoscopy) in the absence of middle ear of mastoid disease. This is seen in superior semicircular canal dehiscence where Tullio phenomenon, vertigo induced by loud sounds, may also be seen.

34. Answer C

There are 5 portions of the temporal bone: the tympanic, mastoid, petrous, zygomatic and squamous. Complications of acute otitis media arise from effects of the infection on structures within the tympanum (perforation, facial palsy, hearing loss, suppurative labyrinthitis etc.), or due to extension of the infection from its origin in the tympanic temporal bone to adjacent sites. Infection can spread to the mastoid portion resulting in the classical mastoid abscess. Less commonly, it can track extra-temporally along structures that insert into the mastoid tip; either along the sternocleidomastoid (Bezold's abscess) or along the posterior belly of the digastric (Citelli's abscess). The infection can spread to the squamous temporal bone and cause an abscess under the temporalis muscle (Luc's abscess) or extend along the zygomatic root causing an abscess over the zygomatic root.

35. Answer B

Blind sac closure of ear involves removal of the posterior ear canal wall along with all of the squamous epithelium of the external auditory canal (EAC) including the tympanic membrane. The most lateral EAC skin is everted and sutured together. The middle ear space is filled with a fat graft/temporalis muscle flap and the Eustachian tube orifice is typically occluded to prevent migration of pathogens from the nasopharynx. Although this is quite a radical option it can be useful in patients with particularly aggressive disease with multiple recurrences. Since the external auditory canal is closed off, air conduction is sacrificed. As such this procedure should be reserved for revision cases in which there is an existing hearing deficit in an ear which is unfavourable for reconstruction with ossiculoplasty.

36. Answer D

Whilst unilateral hearing is sufficient for speech development there is evidence of increased listening effort and difficulty in noisy environments, both of which increase cognitive load. In a deaf child whose parents wish for their child to engage in verbal communication, early aiding to prevent cognitive deprivation of the auditory cortex is important as early as possible. In a patient with microtia, the ability for air conduction aiding will be compromised since there is no outer ear anatomy or ear canal to conduct sound. Pinna reconstruction is usually not recommended before 9 years old, to allow for growth and also allow the child to contribute to management discussions.

37. Answer A

At this age, the best auditory rehabilitation option likely remains the use of a softband bone conduction hearing aid. This can be a challenge for some children and using the input and skills of a multidisciplinary team including speech therapy, audiology, teachers of the deaf and clinical psychologist, combined with good communication with the child's school, are all important. The auditory implant team will be looking at softband use to determine whether the patient is likely to benefit (and will use) an implantable bone conduction aid such as an OSIA or Bonebridge implant. In single-sided deafness such implants are usually offered beyond the patient's current age, although this is a point for individual discussion. In the era of more auditory implant choices, canalplasty for congenital atresia is not usually undertaken in the UK, since the surgery has a high re-stenosis rate and may increase the risk of complications such as a discharging ear.

38. Answer B

Masking is a noise presented to the non-test ear to ensure the tone presented to the test ear is not heard on the opposite side. It is mandatory for determining accurate hearing thresholds in the presence of asymmetrical levels between the two ears and for ascertaining the presence of a conductive hearing loss. In situations in which there is a sizeable conductive component in both ears, it may not be possible to mask effectively at all. This is known as the masking dilemma: the required intensity to mask the non-test ear crosses over to the other ear and invalidates the thresholds. This is the case in this scenario because there is severe otosclerosis causing a likely severe to profound hearing loss (patient is being assessed for cochlear implant) and therefore the volume required to test the non-test ear will need to be very loud and potentially cross over and be picked up by the non-test ear.

39. Answer C

Labyrinthine fistula encountered during surgery increases the risk of developing a dead ear, which is all the more concerning in this patient who is having surgery in her only hearing ear. Whilst continuing to elevate the matrix and covering with temporalis fascia, bone dust and fibrin glue may be appropriate in other circumstances, the safest option for this patient would be to leave a small amount of matrix and return in 6 months in the hope that the cholesteatoma has formed a pearl that can subsequently be removed. MRI scanning is used to monitor disease once all the macroscopic disease has been removed but is not sensitive for cholesteatoma <2 mm. Applying laser to a potential canal fistula would increase the chance of developing a dead ear and obliterating the cavity with residual matrix remaining in situ risks developing a cholesteatoma recurrence.

40. **Answer A**

This patient has had previous surgery with attempt at TORP reconstruction which has not closed the air-bone gap. The mastoids are opacified and likely to be full of scar tissue which may reduce the chance of revision ossiculoplasty surgery being successful. Whilst encouraging use of a softband is a good option, this has usually been tried previously and so may not have been a successful option for this patient. Whilst an OSIA and Bonebridge implant are both potential options, the MDT is likely to want consistent softband use before recommending surgery especially if this child may end up being a poor user of the implant (as with the softband). The best *initial* treatment for *hearing improvement* in this case, given the likely middle ear effusions with conductive hearing loss, is bilateral grommet insertion.

41. **Answer B**

A long history of a discharging left ear and evidence of cholesteatoma on examination means that combined-approach tympanomastoidectomy to remove any residual cholesteatoma sac is the best definitive option for this patient. A cartilage tympanoplasty will prevent further retraction but will not definitively address any trapped residual keratin from the retraction, which could be left behind and lead to recurrence of the cholesteatoma. Instilling trimovate cream to see if the auto-atticotomy cavity/cholesteatoma settles/has been removed completely is an option but it is not the best definitive option for the patient. Offering a hearing aid will not address the underlying issue of a cholesteatoma which will progress without surgical treatment.

42. **Answer B**

A phase II study looking at the use of pentoxifylline and vitamin E in patients with refractory osteoradionecrosis resulted in all patients experiencing a complete recovery in a median of 9 months. Biopsy of the ear canal is necessary to exclude recurrent or synchronous malignancy but this is an investigation or management option rather than a treatment. Lateral temporal bone resection is a treatment for ear canal malignancy.

43. **Answer E**

This patient is presenting with bilateral acute otitis media which is complicated by bony erosions and an epidural abscess. The definitive treatment is surgical treatment with cortical mastoidectomy to obtain source control and help drain the mastoids. A discussion with neurosurgery is an option beforehand but management of an abscess of this size may be non-surgical and resolve with drainage of the mastoid abscess and intravenous antibiotics. Addressing source control with mastoidectomies is the least morbid option. Examination of the ears and grommet insertion may help on the left but the right ear is already discharging and the infection has progressed despite this. Continuing antibiotics is a good option but should be done in conjunction with surgical management.

44. **Answer B**

There is a suggestion of immediate traumatic facial nerve injury with a fracture line transecting the facial nerve canal. Nerve conduction studies are useful to identify the degree of Wallerian degeneration and the benefit of exploring and decompressing the facial nerve. After an injury Wallerian degeneration takes up to 72 hours to occur and therefore performing electroneurography testing prior to 72 hours post injury will potentially give a falsely re-assuring result. Surgery is indicated if there is greater than 90% nerve fibre degeneration on the injured side compared to the unaffected side. Electromyography tests facial muscle function and compares each side of the face. It can be used in cases in which there is greater than 90% nerve fibre degeneration at least 2–3 weeks after the paralysis. Absence of action potentials provides evidence that a patient may benefit from the decompression of the facial nerve.

Audiogram will be useful to verify the presence of a dead ear, which will help in choosing a surgical approach but is not possible in an intubated patient. Waiting until the patient is extubated may result in missing the opportunity to intervene and decompress the nerve.

45. Answer D

This question is about a BIPP reaction in a patient who has had 2 operations on his ears. BIPP reactions often present similarly to a post-operative infection with itching and swelling being key features. Because it is an allergic reaction, prophylactic antibiotics will not help, and whilst removing the packing will alleviate the symptoms, avoiding the BIPP altogether is the best option. In patients having revision surgery alternative packing materials such as a pope wick and topical antibiotics should be considered to avoid this complication.

46. Answer A

Necrotising otitis externa is an increasingly common presentation to ENT. Nuclear medicine scanning has been used either to label white cells or osteoblastic activity but is non-specific and does not necessarily show resolution of changes with resolution of infection. Gallium scans incorporate radioisotopes into white cells and bacteria but there are reports of normal scans found in patients with recurrent disease. Bone scans are very sensitive in making the diagnosis (although positive scans may be found in simple otitis externa) and these do not normalise with resolution of infection so they are not helpful for determining the end of treatment. CT and MRI imaging provide complimentary information. CT is best for the initial diagnosis of bony erosion, whilst MRI can help determine the extent of disease and monitoring response to treatment, as well as distinguishing skull base osteomyelitis from nasopharyngeal carcinoma. Given the symptoms and otomicroscopic findings have resolved, a CRP to ensure no ongoing inflammation is a useful investigation which is cost effective and has no radiation implications.

47. Answer C

In this scenario, the differential diagnosis of hearing loss in association with an upper-respiratory tract infection includes glue ear, acute otitis media, otitis externa or sudden sensorineural hearing loss. In this case the diagnosis is established with the tuning fork tests which are suggestive of a sensorineural hearing loss on the left side. The blocked sensation is a result of hearing loss on that side. In view of the sensorineural hearing loss, answers A, B and C are reasonable options. But, in the absence of any contraindications an oral steroid course is widely accepted as the initial management of choice. Intratympanic steroids may be used in combination with oral steroids or as salvage therapy. (At the time of writing, this treatment dilemma is the subject of a UK multicentre randomised controlled trial, so treatment advice trends may change following the results of this). The patient will need an MRI IAM, but this can be performed at a later date.

48. Answer B

In this scenario, the patient has developed an acute sensorineural hearing loss on the right side. An oral steroid course is the widely accepted initial management for this condition; however, the patient has two relative contraindications to an oral steroid course: uncontrolled diabetes and a gastric ulcer. An intratympanic steroid injection seems more appropriate to prevent the systemic effects of an oral steroid course in this scenario. An expedited endocrinology follow-up is unlikely to rapidly control his deranged glucose especially if he is already on insulin. The most likely cause of his hearing loss is small vessel occlusion as opposed to vasculitis/syphilis or Lyme disease.

49. Answer C

In this scenario the patient is suffering with a right-sided pulsatile tinnitus which is synchronous with his heartbeat. This represents a venous or arterial bruit which is heard on the ipsilateral side. Compression of the right neck would compress the internal jugular vein (IJV) suggesting that this is a venous bruit in proximity to the ear. A dehiscence of the sigmoid sinus within the temporal bone is sometimes seen. In the first instance a CTA/V is warranted to investigate for a vascular anomaly that could account for the symptoms. If this is normal and the symptoms are still persistent, then an MRI can be useful as a second stage. Contrast is essential to establish the anatomy of the vasculature; hence a CT temporal bones alone is insufficient. Pure tone audiogram and MRI IAM is useful for unilateral non-pulsatile tinnitus to investigate for retrocochlear lesions such as a vestibular schwannoma.

50. Answer A

In this scenario, the patient has third window symptoms and signs specifically autophony, Tullio phenomenon and a positive fistula test. This can occur due to any third window of the labyrinth. In this scenario given the history of ear discharge and an ear polyp, the most likely cause is cholesteatoma. Cholesteatoma within the epitympanum is in closest proximity to the lateral semicircular canal; hence this is the correct answer in the scenario.

51. Answer A

In this scenario the patient has signs of a left-sided peripheral vestibular irritation causing left-beating nystagmus. This could result from labyrinthitis, vestibular neuronitis, or Meniere's disease. Stroke could also cause these symptoms but is unlikely in this age-group and typically causes a central pattern of nystagmus. In vestibular neuronitis the hearing is preserved since the patient only suffers with vertigo. It is unlikely for Meniere's disease to cause episodes of vertigo lasting >12 hours.

52. Answer C

In this scenario, the patient has acute left vestibular failure. On examination you would expect to see a spontaneous horizontal-rotational nystagmus with the fast phase beating towards the healthy ear, which would be the right ear in this scenario. Alexander's law states that a second- or third-degree nystagmus will enhance on gaze deviation in the direction of the fast phase.

53. Answer A

In this scenario the patient has significant right Meniere's disease which is impacting his life. He has little residual hearing left on the affected side. The options for treatment include A-D but given that there is no residual hearing, ablative options including intratympanic gentamicin or labyrinthectomy can be considered. He is keen for the most definitive solution; hence labyrinthectomy is recommended. Vestibular neurectomy are rarely undertaken in the UK and require a neurosurgical approach as opposed to a labyrinthectomy which can be performed via a transmastoid approach.

54. Answer A

In this scenario the patient has developed left-sided BPPV following trauma. The treatment is the Epley manoeuvre. This follows the description in A, starting by turning the head of the patient to the contralateral side to correct the otolith position within the labyrinth.

55. Answer A

In this scenario, the symptoms are suggestive of a left-sided third window of the inner ear. The symptoms are typical of left-sided superior semicircular canal dehiscence (SSCD). Patients with this condition have the defect identified on CT imaging, but there is a significant number of patients who have this dehiscence present with no symptoms. Patients do have a supranormal bone conduction on the ipsilateral side with an apparent ipsilateral conductive element. However, Cervical VEMP testing is most useful at identifying a functional dehiscence because the waveforms have a lower threshold and high amplitude on the affected side. Patients who have a significantly impaired quality of life with radiological and audiometric consistent results can be offered resurfacing or plugging of the affected superior semicircular canal.

56. Answer C

In this scenario the patient's symptoms and radiology suggest a left-sided superior semicircular canal dehiscence. This would result in third window signs on the left side, including a positive fistula test on the left. SSCD causes a supranormal bone conduction on the affected side and thus an 'apparent' conductive loss. This would result in the Weber going to the left side. The Rinne on the right would be unaffected. Typically, due to the third window, a tuning fork placed on bony prominences like the elbow or ankle are heard in the affected ear—in this case the left side. The Dix-Hallpike test is for BPPV which would be normal in this scenario.

57. Answer C

Active middle ear implants are surgically implanted devices that stimulate the ossicular chain or round window membrane via a floating mass transducer and appropriate coupler. They may be used as part of the treatment of certain patients with sensorineural hearing loss as well as for conductive or mixed hearing loss. These patients must have stable hearing thresholds to avoid falling out of criteria and the device being rendered obsolete.

58. Answer E

Temporal bone trauma can result in damage to either an ossicular joint or the individual ossicles themselves. Joint dislocation is the most common pattern of injury with dislocation of the incudo-stapedial joint being the most frequently found at the time of surgical exploration. Incudo-mallear joint dislocation has been reported as the most common site for dislocation on imaging; however, this is likely because the incudo-stapedial joint is less easily assessed on CT scan. Ossicular fractures are much less common.

59. Answer D

A meta-analysis by Yu et al. in 2013 showed that PORP has significantly improved post-operative hearing outcomes along with a significantly lower rate of extrusion at long-term follow-up. The use of PORP leads to a closure of the air-bone gap to less than 20 dB in over 70% of patients whilst case series using TORP between the footplate and TM noted post-operative mean ABG ≤20 dB in approximately half to two thirds of patients. Successful air-bone gap closure is considered <20 dB in the literature. Surgical results from ossiculoplasty prostheses may deteriorate over time.

60. Answer D

Tympanoplasty can be divided into five types according to the Wullstein classification. This would be a type IV reconstruction.

> **Wullstein classification:**
>
> Type I: Myringoplasty
>
> Type II: TM to incus/malleus remnant or restoration of lever mechanism (ISJ erosion)
>
> Type III: TM to stapes suprastructure
>
> Type IV: a repair when the stapes foot plate is mobile but the superstructure is missing. The resulting middle ear will consist of the Eustachian tube and hypo-tympanum. Fascia is used to create a round window baffle
>
> Type V: Fenestration procedure e.g LSCC

61. Answer D

Hyrtl's fissure (tympanomeningeal fissure) is a congenital infralabyrinthine fissure in the foetal petrous temporal bone and is usually closed by the normal progression of ossification in the 24th week of gestation. It occasionally persists and has been reported as a rare cause of CSF otorrhoea and meningitis.

62. Answer D

Many surgeons will wait until a child is 7 years or older to perform a myringoplasty although practice does vary considerably. A meta-analysis demonstrated that the children with abnormal contralateral ear findings were more likely to have an unsuccessful outcome following a myringoplasty and the authors suggested surgery may best be delayed until contralateral otitis media with effusion had settled (Hardman et al. Tympanoplasty for chronic tympanic membrane perforation in children: systematic review and meta-analysis. *Otology & Neurotology* 2015; 36(5): 796–804). Evidence surrounding the success of myringoplasty in patients with prior adenoidectomy is conflicting.

63. Answer E

Tenderness of the masticatory muscles is seen the majority of patients with TMJ dysfunction, with tenderness of the lateral pterygoid in 85% of patients; 67% of patients had joint tenderness with 38% having crepitus on examination. MRI can demonstrate an effusion or joint changes but rarely contributes to the diagnosis.

64. Answer D

Pseudomonas is the most common organism in CSOM and can be difficult to eradicate due to biofilm production and the presence of persister cells. *Staphylococcus aureus* and *Streptococcus pneumoniae* may also cause CSOM. Other causative bacteria include *Haemophilus influenzae*, *Moraxella catarrhalis*, Proteus spp.,

Peptostreptococcus spp. and Prevotella spp. In immunosuppressed patients fungal infections including Candida and Aspergillus may be present.

65. Answer B

In this scenario, the symptoms suggest auditory neuropathy spectrum disorder (ANSD), a specific form of hearing impairment in which the patient can hear the sound of speech but has difficulties understanding the words. It is caused by auditory dyssynchrony/abnormal neural synchrony; i.e. the loudness of sound is relatively well perceived, but the synchronisation of acoustic signals is not adequate to evoke an ABR, or to elicit the stapedial reflex, or to suppress the contralateral transient evoked otoacoustic emissions (TOAEs). In the case of abnormal hair cell function we would not expect to see normal OAEs. In language development disorders, you would not expect to see normal pure tone audiometry with abnormal or absent ABR.

66. Answer E

This is a Sadé grade 4 retraction according to the table 1.1:

Table 1.1

	Pars Flaccida (Tos)	Pars Tensa (Sadé)
Grade 1:	Attic dimpling	Mild retraction
Grade 2:	Retraction onto malleus neck	Onto ISJ
Grade 3:	Scutum erosion	Onto promontory but non-adhesive
Grade 4:	Cholesteatoma	Adherent to promontory

67. Answer D

Treacher Collins or mandibulofacial dysostosis arises following abnormal differentiation of the first and second pharyngeal arches. Mutations in other genes (*POLR1B, POLR1C, POLR1D*) have been identified. Several features are commonly identified with the syndrome: downslanting palpebral fissures (89–100%); malar or zygomatic complex hypoplasia (81–97%); conductive hearing loss (83–92%); atresia of EAC (68–71%); coloboma (54–69%); tracheostomy in neonates (12–18%). However, intellectual disability is unusual. Most children require multiple operations until early adulthood. It is important to ensure an echocardiogram is performed to rule out cardiac abnormalities.

68. Answer E

The correct answer is furuncle. While otitis externa is a potential possibility, the intensity of the pain described in the vignette aligns more closely with a furuncle. These localised infections usually involve a single hair follicle or sweat gland within the outer third of the cartilaginous EAC, resulting in a painful boil or pustule. Conversely, otitis externa involves a broader infection affecting the entire ear canal. The vignette does not mention visual loss, making temporal arteritis (giant cell arteritis) less probable; however, clinically it would be prudent to assess for a temporal artery pulse in a patient of this age. Temporal arteritis can also manifest with severe pain in the temporal region and jaw claudication. Contact dermatitis, a Type IV hypersensitivity reaction, arises from exposure to allergens or irritants, leading to symptoms like redness, itching and fluid-filled bumps upon skin contact. First branchial cleft anomalies emerge near the external ear, appearing as cysts, sinuses or fistulas, causing intermittent drainage, infections and discomfort. However, this diagnosis is less likely given the patient's age.

69. Answer C

In this scenario, the patient's initial symptoms of acute vertigo lasting 2–3 days with the absence of any hearing symptoms suggest acute vestibular failure (vestibular neuronitis/acute peripheral vestibulopathy). The following episodes of brief positional vertigo are typical for benign paroxysmal positional vertigo (BPPV) which can occur in association with other labyrinthine disease such as vestibular neuronitis or Meniere's disease.

70. Answer C

The most characteristic clinical finding with sudden unilateral loss of vestibular function is spontaneous peripheral vestibular nystagmus which is characteristically horizontal with a torsional component. An acute loss of peripheral vestibular function results in a slow vestibular-induced drift of the eyes in the same direction as the lesion which is the left side in this case. This drift is interrupted by rapid saccadic eye movements in the opposite direction, towards the healthy ear. In acute severe cases, the nystagmus is initially present with optic fixation but, in milder cases and during recovery, there will be no visible nystagmus with optic fixation, and it is not until the optic fixation has been removed that the nystagmus will be present.

71. Answer B

Granular myringitis is characterised by inflammation of the external ear canal and tympanic membrane, presenting with symptoms such as itching, pain and discharge. The tympanic membrane may appear reddened, swollen and covered with granulation tissue. Potential complications include tympanosclerosis or tympanic membrane perforation. It can be distinguished from other conditions like otitis externa by the presence of granulation tissue on the tympanic membrane, as well as the absence of fungal elements. Aetiological factors include bacterial or viral infections, irritants (like chronic use of ear drops) and fungal infections. Contributing host factors such as immune compromise might also play a role. Histologically, granular myringitis shows hyperplasia of the epithelial lining, infiltration of inflammatory cells and the presence of granulation tissue. The tissue changes are most prominent in the external ear canal and the tympanic membrane.

It is important to distinguish from bullous myringitis, which involves painful blisters on the tympanic membrane. It can be mistaken for granular myringitis due to similar symptoms, but the presence of blisters is the distinguishing factor. It is commonly associated with *Mycoplasma pneumoniae*, *Streptococcus pneumoniae*, and *Haemophilus influenzae*. Bullous myringitis is differentiated from acute otitis media by the presence of vesicles or blisters on the eardrum, which are usually not seen in otitis media. Fungal infections of the ear can present with similar symptoms to myringitis, including pain, itching and discharge. Otomycosis often results in a fungal overgrowth in the ear canal, but the tympanic membrane itself may not be affected; furthermore, no black conidiophores or white filamentous hyphae are seen on examination, making this unlikely. Tympanosclerosis involves the formation of calcified deposits on the tympanic membrane and ankylosis of the ossicles due to repeated infections or inflammation. It can cause changes in the appearance of the tympanic membrane, but it lacks the characteristic inflammation and granulation tissue seen in myringitis.

72. Answer D

In this clinical scenario, several potential diagnoses need to be considered, including keratosis obturans, EAC cholesteatoma, necrotising otitis externa (NOE), squamous cell carcinoma (SCC) of the EAC and exostoses. These conditions share common features such as ear pain and infection of the external ear canal.

Exostoses are characterised by the development of smooth lamellar bone growths and are often associated with cold water swimming. Given the absence of this association in the patient's history, it makes exostoses an unlikely diagnosis, effectively excluding Option A.

NOE is typically seen in individuals who are diabetic or immunocompromised. However, the patient in this case does not have these risk factors, and the absence of a facial nerve palsy further reduces the likelihood of advanced NOE or SCC of the EAC, leading to the exclusion of Options B and C.

The two most probable differential diagnoses remaining are keratosis obturans and EAC cholesteatoma. However, a crucial distinguishing feature in keratosis obturans is the absence of bony necrosis or sequestration of underlying bone. Keratosis obturans is typically managed conservatively with lifelong microsuction (Option E). On the other hand, EAC cholesteatoma often requires surgical resection, often via a canal wall down procedure to remove the sequestered bone and ulcerated overlying skin, followed by reconstruction of the canal and split skin grafting (Option D).

Most cases of EAC cholesteatoma occur unilaterally, and they are more common in the elderly population, leading to chronic unilateral dull pain due to the invasion of squamous tissue into a localised area of periostitis in the canal wall. Keratosis obturans can also be associated with sinusitis or bronchiectasis in a significant percentage of children and adults, and bilateral occurrences are more common in children.

73. Answer C

Necrotising otitis externa is the likely pathology, risk factors for this pathology include immunocompromise or diabetes mellitus, elderly age, external auditory canal trauma, granulomatosis with polyangiitis, and previous radiotherapy. Although this pathology is often referred to as malignant otitis externa, the aetiology is solely infectious and inflammatory. Surgical debridement is not routinely undertaken and is occasionally employed due to the lack of improvement following conservative treatment. There is also some belief that surgery to obtain tissue for histology and/or microbiology is beneficial but there is no evidence it improves long-term outcomes of facial palsy recovery. A survey of current practice undertaken of otolaryngologists in the UK suggests 50% used monotherapy and 37% used dual therapy. With regards to the causative organism, the most common organism in patients who are diabetic is *Pseudomonas aeruginosa* not *Aspergillus* species; however, *S. aureus* and MRSA are more prevalent in non-diabetic patients, making Option C the correct answer.

74. Answer A

The vignette is describing 'surfer's ear' or exostoses of the external ear canal. Although the exact mechanism for these is not fully understood, it is thought that cold water stimulates reflex vasodilatation triggering bone growth by increasing osteoblastic activity in susceptible individuals, possibly to protect the EAC or tympanic membrane from the cold. This process results in excessive lamellar bone formation (Option A). The incidence in the general population is estimated to be 5%. The common differential are osteomas (Option B), these after often solitary bony growths within the EAC and are composed of either compact, spongy or mixed bone. The former contains a Haversian system, whereas the spongy type contains trabecular bone with marrow. Exostoses are not associated with sequestration of bone; this is seen in external canal cholesteatoma (Option C). Additionally, these lesions are benign, and Option E suggests a malignant process; SCC is the most common EAC malignancy, responsible for an estimated 50%. Option D is describing keratosis obliterans, in which accumulation of keratin results in remoulding of the EAC and hyperplasia of the epithelium.

75. Answer A

In this scenario, the patient's episodic dizziness, headache, photophobia and phono-phobia suggest a diagnosis of vestibular migraine. The absence of hearing loss is helpful in differentiating vestibular migraine from Meniere's disease in which a sustained low-frequency unilateral hearing loss may be detected. However, to confirm the diagnosis and assess the vestibular system, the most appropriate investigation is still an MRI of the brain to exclude any central pathology. Increased time constants may be seen on rotation testing. Abnormal posturography is present in around one third and a canal paresis on caloric testing in around a quarter. Vestibular evoked myogenic potential (VEMP) abnormalities are non-specific and variable.

76. Answer B

Table 1.2

Tuning fork (Hz)	Rinne test result	Air-bone gap (dB)
256	negative	>15
512	negative	>25
1024	negative	>35

The principle of the Rinne test is to compare perceptions of bone conduction (BC) and air conduction (AC) sounds. To achieve this, placing a vibrating tuning fork over the mastoid bone will test the former (BC), whilst placing the fork—so that the tines line up—lateral to the external auditory canal (EAC) will test the latter (AC). A positive 'normal' test is declared when AC is heard louder than BC, whereas a negative 'abnormal' test result occurs when BC is heard louder than AC. Two commonly adopted methods are undertaken: either by asking the patient to identify if the sound is heard louder when delivered through AC or via BC; or, alternatively, by the timed threshold technique whereby the tuning fork is initially placed over the mastoid bone, and once the patient indicates they no longer are able to hear it, the tuning fork is moved lateral to the EAC. Should the patient still hear the sound of the tuning fork the test is considered to be positive. The frequency of the tuning fork used in the Rinne test to detect conductive hearing loss depends on the size of the air-bone gap (see Table 1.2).

Incorrect answers:

A Testing with both 256 Hz and 512 Hz are positive

C Testing with both 256 Hz and 512 Hz are likely negative, but positive with 1024 Hz

D Testing with both 256 Hz and 512 Hz negative, but possibly positive with 1024 Hz

E Negative with all three

77. Answer E

A Sadé Grade 3 is defined as retraction of the tympanic membrane onto the promontory, but not adherent as evidenced by inflation on Valsalva manoeuvre. The distinction between Sadé Grade 3 and Grade 4 retraction is often challenging and usually confirmed intra-operatively by distinguishing if the tympanic membrane is truly adherent to the promontory.

78. Answer D

All of these structures must be considered when performing a translabyrinthine approach to the CPA. The initial part of the operation is an extended mastoidectomy in which, in addition to a cortical mastoidectomy, the middle and posterior fossa dura and sigmoid sinus are skeletonised. The skeletonisation of structures allows retraction to increase working space for bone and tumour removal.

A labyrinthectomy is then performed in which all semi-circular canals are drilled out. The vestibule is identified as an important landmark, the floor of the labyrinth being the roof of the internal auditory meatus (IAM). The neuroepithelium in the floor of the labyrinth is preserved as a marker of the position of the superior and inferior vestibular nerve canals later in the procedure to aid in identification of the IAM. The cochlea is not routinely removed unless an intracochlear tumour is also present. If the cochlea is drilled out, then the petrous carotid artery is seen anterior and inferior to the basal turn.

The vertical facial nerve is then skeletonised to allow for safe retrofacial dissection towards the petrous apex. The jugular bulb is then found inferiorly to mark the inferior limit of the dissection. The cochlea aqueduct (containing the perilymphatic duct draining perilymph into the CSF of the posterior cranial fossa subarachnoid space) is encountered superior to the jugular bulb. The egress of CSF is helpful to the surgeon since it decompresses the posterior fossa necessitating less retraction. Drilling between the jugular bulb and cochlear aqueduct will take the surgeon to the lower cranial nerves which can be inadvertently damaged.

The bone between the bulb (inferiorly) and middle fossa dura (superiorly) is then removed from the posterior fossa dura on a broad front to identify the internal auditory meatus which runs from deep posteriorly (posterior fossa dura) to superficial anteriorly (floor of vestibule). The IAM is then skeletonised and opened to identify the superior and inferior vestibular nerves, facial nerve and cochlear nerve.

79. Answer C

This patient has a non-contrast MRI scan showing likely bilateral vestibular schwannomas. NF2-related schwannomatosis (NF2) is characterised by bilateral vestibular schwannomas, the symptoms of which are tinnitus, hearing loss and balance dysfunction. The average age of onset is 18–24 years. Almost all affected individuals will have bilateral vestibular schwannomas by 30 years old. They may also present with schwannomas affecting other cranial nerves, meningiomas or ependymomas, or subcapsular cataracts.

To complete the radiological work-up for this patient, post-contrast MRI imaging of entire brain is required to assess for enhancement of the facial nerve, thus distinguishing a facial from a vestibular schwannoma, and to assess for other intracranial tumours (meningiomas, ependymomas and schwannomas of other cranial nerves). Whole spine post-contrast MRI imaging is also required to look for spinal meningiomas and ependymomas.

A referral to clinical genetics will be required after radiological work-up is complete. NF2 is inherited in an autosomal dominant manner: 50% of individuals with NF2 will have an affected parent and 50% will have NF2 as a result of a *de novo* mutation. All affected individuals will have genetic testing. At-risk family members are identified and offered annual neurological examination and annual MRI brain scans, audiology and ophthalmology examinations from the age of 12 years.

Bevacizumab (Avastin) is a monoclonal IgG antibody which inhibits angiogenesis by binding vascular endothelial growth factor (VEGF). It is used in NF2 patients to control growth in schwannomas exhibiting >80% increase in volume in 12 months or for whom there is an imminent threat to neurological function. Assessment for treatment is via specialist regional NF2 centres. It is usually given every 2–3 weeks intravenously. It is associated with bleeding risk and clotting issues, hypertension and proteinuria and hence is not indicated for sporadic vestibular schwannomas. In this case there is no imminent threat to neurological function and growth over 12 months has not been ascertained; therefore, current referral would be inappropriate.

80. Answer B

This patient is presenting with a life-threatening neurosurgical emergency. The priority is to treat the hydrocephalus and thus relieve pressure on the brain. A lumbar puncture in the emergency department may be used to sample CSF and assess the opening pressure; however, that will not provide definitive hydrocephalus management. Emergency VP shunt insertion overnight will allow for CSF diversion while a definitive plan is made for tumour excision.

A large vestibular schwannoma, as in this case, exerts pressure on the brainstem. This patient's hearing and balance have deteriorated over several years. Facial numbness in large tumours occurs due to trigeminal nerve irritation. Severe imbalance and decreased level of consciousness is seen with a critical rise in intracranial pressure. Tumour excision overnight is not recommended because surgical planning and the involvement of a specialist skull base (neurosurgical and ENT) team is required. Definitive surgery should be planned for the next available opportunity.

There are four surgical routes to access a tumour within the CPA: translabyrinthine, retrosigmoid, middle cranial fossa and transpromontorial approaches. In this case the translabyrinthine route would be preferred since it provides direct tumour access without the need for brain retraction, early identification of the facial nerve (which remains fully functional in this patient) and since hearing is already lost. A retrosigmoid approach is also appropriate for large tumours (and can offer hearing preservation if not already lost); however, the need for cerebellar retraction in this case makes it less attractive. The middle cranial fossa approach is utilised primarily for small tumours within the internal auditory canal and would not be appropriate in this case. Similarly, the transcanal endoscopic transpromontorial approach can be used to treat small tumours in the internal auditory canal (IAC); however, is not widely practised and would not be suitable in this case.

81. Answer B

All of the options are lesions that can be found in the cerebellopontine angle (CPA) and show enhancement on post-contrast MRI. By far the most common lesion involving the CPA is vestibular schwannoma (80%) followed by meningioma (10%). Vestibular schwannomas classically primarily involve the IAC causing enlargement, then grow into the CPA. Meningiomas can also involve the IAC by extending into it from an adjacent location. They are classically broad based on the petrous bone with dural tails and often show calcification. CT scanning shows enlargement of the IAC in vestibular schwannoma and hyperostosis of adjacent bone in meningioma.

Schwannomas of the facial nerve can be challenging to distinguish from vestibular schwannomas. Careful examination of asymmetrical enhancement of the geniculate ganglion and labyrinthine facial nerve on post-contrast MRI scanning, in addition to a high index of suspicion in patients presenting with early facial nerve symptoms, are important features of the diagnosis. CPA ependymomas are uncommon lesions usually seen in children. They displace surrounding tissues and the brainstem and so the most common presenting symptoms are those of raised intracranial pressure. The majority of posterior fossa ependymomas arise from the fourth ventricle and may extend through the foramina of Luschka and Magendie.

Ependymomas are heterogenous on CT and MRI imaging with areas of necrosis, calcification, cystic change and haemorrhage frequently seen. Metastases must be considered in view of the patient's past medical history. The most common sites of origin for metastatic deposits in the CPA are breast, lung and malignant melanoma. Metastases behave aggressively and would be less likely in this case due to the patient's long period of remission.

82. Answer B

The vertical crest, commonly known as Bill's bar, separates the superior compartment of the internal auditory meatus (IAM) into an anterior compartment containing the facial nerve and nervus intermedius, and posterior compartment containing the superior vestibular nerve.

The falciform or transverse crest divides the IAM into superior and inferior compartments. The inferior compartment contains the cochlear nerve anteriorly and inferior vestibular nerve posteriorly.

The aide memoire '7-up' (facial nerve superiorly) and 'Coke down' (cochlear nerve inferiorly) with both lying anteriorly in the IAM can be employed. The position of the nerve within the IAM is crucial to protect the facial and sometimes cochlear nerve,

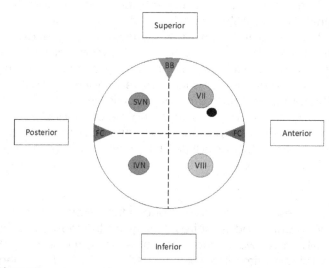

Figure 1.4 Bill's Bar Diagram.

during removal of vestibular schwannomas arising from either the superior or inferior vestibular nerves.

83. Answer C

In cases of facial nerve injury, it takes 72 hours for Wallerian degeneration (the denervation of neural fibres) to occur. Before 72 hours the fibres remain physiologically intact, although non-functional volitionally. This patient is presenting 3 days after the onset of weakness and therefore we can assume that Wallerian degeneration has occurred.

ENoG is used to evaluate the integrity of the facial nerve and the most useful test to predict recovery at this point. The procedure involves electrical stimulation of the facial nerve at the stylomastoid foramen and measurement of the motor response at the ipsilateral naso-labial fold. ENoG compares the neurophysiological response of the normal side to the abnormal side. Nerve fibre degeneration leads to a decrease or loss of the compound muscle action potential (CMAP). The amplitude of the CMAP on the affected side is compared to the CMAP of the unaffected side and expressed as a percentage (amplitude of the paralysed side divided by the amplitude of the normal side). ENoG can be used from 72 hours to 21 days post injury and is usually repeated at intervals of 3 to 5 days until a trend is observed thus informing the decision regarding the need for surgical intervention.

After the onset of an acute facial palsy, before the lesion has become complete, EMG can be used to detect the presence of voluntary motor action potentials. A facial motor unit consists of a facial motor neuron and all the muscle fibres innervated by it. A needle electrode in a facial muscle measures the amplitude and duration of the facial motor action potential produced on attempted movement. This is useful in traumatic cases because, if present, it proves that the nerve has not been transected. In this case EMG would be most helpful 2–3 weeks after the onset of weakness and loss of nerve excitability. Pathological spontaneous activity in the form of fibrillation potentials or positive sharp waves is a sign of facial nerve degeneration. After 4–6 weeks, polyphasic reinnervation potentials are signs of muscle reinnervation.

Stapedial (acoustic) reflex testing can aid in the localisation of a facial nerve injury but not the likelihood of recovery. The absence of the stapedial reflex is expected in intratemporal facial nerve lesions arising proximal to the stapedial muscle. Return of the reflex is an early sign of recovery that usually precedes the recovery of facial movement. PTA and tympanometry should be performed in all cases of facial weakness to aid investigation of possible causes of facial weakness (e.g. cholesteatoma). MRI scanning can be used to assess for structural lesions and gadolinium enhancement of the facial nerve has been described in Bell's palsy and Ramsay-Hunt syndrome; however, the association between levels of enhancement and recovery is not well understood.

84. Answer D

In this case the patient is keen to prevent any further deterioration in her facial function. We have no information as to the previous growth of the facial schwannoma, and so continued surveillance scanning to assess the rate of growth may also be a reasonable answer; however, it is not an option here.

Resection of the tumour will inevitably result in a complete facial weakness (House-Brackmann grade 6) and the best outcome possible with facial reanimation is a House-Brackmann grade 3. Resection is therefore reserved until facial function has deteriorated to a House-Brackmann grade 4 or worse and primary nerve grafting performed. The type of grafting performed is dependent on the size and location of the facial schwannoma.

Stereotactic radiosurgery is a treatment aiming to halt any further growth of the facial schwannoma. However, in view of the patient's young age and good hearing, and the fact that the treatment cannot be repeated, this would be the best option *should the patient be sure she does not wish to undergo surgical intervention at any point.*

Decompression of the facial nerve aims to provide space for the facial schwannoma to grow. Because in this case it is centred on the geniculate ganglion, the middle fossa approach would be the best surgical approach. Transmastoid decompression would be used for a schwannoma affecting the horizonal or vertical facial nerve.

85. Answer A

The most common complication of translabyrinthine resection of vestibular schwannoma is CSF leak. This occurs in approximately 10-15% of cases. The main risk of CSF leak is meningitis; therefore a prompt review with neurological examination is always required. If there are clinical signs of meningism then a lumbar puncture is undertaken with the aim of isolating an organism to target treatment and CT head performed.

Intraoperatively, after tumour removal, conduits for possible CSF leak are obstructed: open mastoid air cells are waxed, the Eustachian tube and middle ear are obliterated with muscle and the surgical cavity is packed with abdominal fat. In some centres a lumbar drain is inserted pre-operatively and left in situ for several days post-operatively to decrease CSF pressure and therefore risk of leak.

CSF leakage can occur directly from the wound site or via the Eustachian tube presenting as unilateral nasal discharge. If there is any clinical uncertainty fluid can be collected and sent for B2 transferrin analysis. In this particular case the leak is low volume via the wound site and so a mattress suture to the leakage site under aseptic conditions is the most appropriate next step in the management of this stable patient. Placement of a lumbar subarachnoid drain may be considered if leakage continued. If this was unsuccessful or if the patient was meningitic then a return to theatre for formal review of the surgical cavity, which may include repacking the cavity with fat, and a multi-layered watertight closure would be required.

In the event of CSF leakage via the nose re-exploration and repacking of the Eustachian tube and middle ear may be required. Blind sac closure of the ear canal is often performed concurrently (eversion of the skin of the lateral ear canal and removal of medial ear canal skin, tympanic membrane, malleus and incus) to seal the cavity. Because the patient has had a translabyrinthine approach he will have no ipsilateral hearing. Endoscopic closure of the Eustachian tube via the nasopharynx is an alternative treatment for CSF rhinorrhoea after the translabyrinthine approach.

86. Answer D

This young patient presents with a paraganglioma. Paragangliomas are slowly growing, usually benign neoplasms, which arise from extra-adrenal paraganglionic tissue derived from neural crest cells. In the head and neck region, parasympathetic-associated paragangliomas are located in four primary sites: the carotid bifurcation, jugular bulb, tympanic plexus and vagal ganglia. Only 5% of head and neck paragangliomas secrete catecholamines. Familial occurrence of paragangliomas is well recognised and is caused by mutations in the succinate dehydrogenase (SDH) subunit genes. This patient requires full radiological, endocrine and genetic work-up before discussion at a specialist multidisciplinary team meeting. A biopsy is not required unless there is diagnostic uncertainty after full work-up and MDT review. The vascularity of the lesion must be considered prior to any biopsy.

Radiologically, CT identifies bony erosion and post-contrast enhanced MRI scan shows small haemorrhages producing T1 hyperintensity (salt) and hypointense areas from flow voids (pepper). Full body scanning is required to assess for the presence of multiple paragangliomas, the gold standard is DOTATATE PET-CT, but full body MRI scanning is also used. Plasma metanephrine analysis needs to be performed with appropriate onward referral to endocrinology if positive. Genetic testing for mutations associated with hereditary paraganglioma and pheochromocytoma (PGL/PCC) syndrome (e.g. SDH genes, *VHL, NF1, MAX* etc.) is undertaken.

Patients with *SDHD* mutations are predisposed to the development of multifocal paragangliomas and those with *SDHB* mutations are at increased risk of malignant paraganglioma. Familial paraganglioma is inherited in an autosomal dominant manner and so genetic testing is also offered to all high-risk family members.

87. Answer C

Michel deformity (complete labyrinthine aplasia) is the absence of the cochlea, vestibule and semi-circular canals. Since there is no inner ear development cochlear implantation is not possible. The only option for audiological rehabilitation in this case is an auditory brainstem implant (ABI). An ABI bypasses the cochlear nerve to electrically stimulate second-order neurons in the cochlear nucleus using a multichannel surface array. ABI can aid in the interpretation of environmental sounds, but open-set speech discrimination cannot be achieved.

A common cavity deformity is one in which there is a single chamber representing the cochlea and vestibule with the IAC entering at its centre. Although theoretically the nerve within the common cavity contains both cochlear and vestibular nerve fibres, it is not possible to determine the percentage of cochlear fibres. Behavioural audiometric responses or aided language development are therefore important to confirm the existence of cochlear fibres. If they are presumed to be present a cochlear implant can be performed using a non-modiolar (straight) electrode positioned on the circumferential wall of the common cavity providing contact with the neural tissue.

Patients with enlarged vestibular aqueduct (EVA) (midpoint between the posterior labyrinth and operculum >1.5 mm) in the presence of a normal cochlea, vestibule and semi-circular canals can undergo cochlear implantation. These patients typically present with stepwise sensorineural hearing loss after minor head trauma.

Incomplete partition represents a group of cochlear malformations. They are subdivided into three groups (IP I–III), all of which all can undergo cochlear implantation but carry a risk of CSF gusher.

In IP-I the entire modiolus and interscalar septa is missing and the vestibule is grossly dilated.

In IP-II the cochlea has only 1.5 turns (Mondini malformation refers to IPII in association with EVA and a dilated vestibule).

In IP-III the interscalar septa is present but the modiolus is absent leading to a corkscrew appearance. The lamina cribrosa separating the basal turn of the cochlea and the fundus of the internal auditory canal (IAC) is absent, resulting in a CSF gusher during CI surgery and a high chance of electrode misplacement into the IAC. It is also referred to as X-linked stapes gusher and is caused by mutations in the *POU3F4* gene.

88. Answer C

This scenario is pointing towards the possibility of enlarged vestibular aqueduct (EVA), which is associated with a progressive sensorineural hearing loss. Vestibular disturbances in EVA, whilst less common, can arise. Mutations in the *SLC26A4* gene can cause EVA as well as Pendred's syndrome, which is also associated with EVA. Thyroid function tests could reveal hypothyroidism in the context of Pendred's syndrome. However, this would not confirm the presence of EVA, nor would option A, B or E. The best definitive test to diagnose EVA in this scenario is CT temporal bones. It is very important to identify EVA pre-operatively, since this has implications on electrode choice in the context of cochlear implantation, as well as counselling regarding chances of post-operative residual hearing preservation.

89. Answer E

The aim to preserve residual hearing is a standard of care in modern day cochlear implantation surgery. This refers to maintaining a patient's pre-operative low-frequency hearing (where present), in those with a ski-slope type hearing loss, such as this patient. 'Soft surgery' is a term referring to the techniques a surgeon can use to improve the chances of hearing preservation. These include non-surgical (e.g. parenteral steroid administration peri-operatively) and surgical considerations, ranging from choice of electrode, type of approach (via delicate opening of the round window membrane vs cochleostomy, careful drilling of the promontory with a low-speed drill), ensuring no suctioning of perilymph nor allowing any blood to enter the cochlea upon opening of the round window, and slow insertion of the electrode. The use of perioperative or intraoperative antibiotics is not in itself connected with hearing preservation.

90. Answer E

Cochlear implant complications can be classified into medical complications, soft failures and hard failures. Medical complications include infection, seroma, abscess, wound breakdown and flap problems (e.g. thickness). 'Soft failures' arise in the context of a device passing the manufacturer's integrity tests, but the patient continues to suffer from non-auditory aversive symptoms, interrupted function and worsening speech intelligibility. When device or hardware failure is identified in testing, this is termed 'hard failure' and usually requires revision surgery/re-implantation. This particular question pertains to electrode migration. Some authors attribute new bone growth or head trauma as potential causes. In this scenario, the surgery was uncomplicated and full insertion was confirmed on intraoperative testing. Options A, B and C would not offer information that would change the patient's management at this stage. The correct answer is E: during switch-on and mapping, the audiologist may be able to deactivate the extracochlear electrodes and follow up the patient closely. Option D would be a consideration if the patient's outcomes remained poor, despite audiological optimisation.

91. Answer C

The wording in this question is very important: choose the "best definitive treatment". The history and investigations support acute otitis media with intra- and extra-cranial complications. Subperiosteal mastoid collection should warrant surgical intervention in the form of cortical mastoidectomy with grommet insertion (as best *definitive* management), especially given the persistently elevated inflammatory markers. This would also allow for pus and tissue samples to be sent for microbiological analysis (microscopy, culture and sensitivity [MC&S], acid fast bacilli [AFB] testing, fungal cultures) to target antimicrobial therapy, especially given the plan for medical management of the small intra-cerebral abscess. The fact that he has recently returned from overseas travel should alert to the possibility of mycobacterial infection, or other atypical pathology. Therefore, whilst Option A should already be instigated, it is not the single best definitive treatment, nor are Options B, D or E.

92. Answer D

The patient in this scenario probably has Goldenhar syndrome (hemifacial microsomia), which is associated with microtia/anotia and aural atresia, as well as ossicular malformations. It is a frequently occurring syndrome in FRCS examinations. There are various grading classifications for microtia. Using the Marx classification, this patient appears to have grade 3 microtia, with evidence of 'peanut ear' (Grade 1—auricle slightly smaller but all subunits present, Grade 2—auricle smaller than Grade 1 with some subunits underdeveloped or absent, Grade 3—small superior cartilage remnant with anteriorly deflected lobule, Grade 4—anotia). The Jahrsdoerfer grading is a 10-point scoring system used as a predictor of favourable outcomes from surgery. Points are allocated as follows: present stapes (2), patent oval window (1), normal round window (1), normal facial nerve (1), incus-stapes connection (1), malleus-incus complex present (1), mastoid well pneumatised (1), normal middle ear space (1). This patient's abnormal incus and microtia gives her a score of 8, Option D.

93. Answer E

This is a scenario of an acute temporal bone fracture in a patient who is intubated and ventilated, with potential CSF leak. There is no strong evidence for commencement of prophylactic broad-spectrum IV antibiotics in the context of CSF leak. The fact remains that the patient has an otic capsule-involving temporal bone fracture, which has a higher likelihood of facial nerve injury compared to otic capsule-sparing fractures. ENoG and EMG testing may be useful in determining prognosis in facial nerve injury. EMG can detect fibrillations from denervated nerve after 2 weeks, whilst ENoG is useful after 72 hours post-injury (when Wallerian degeneration occurs). Therefore, neither Option B nor C is relevant in this acute setting. Option D will not change the current management of this patient. This leaves Option E, which will enable a definitive diagnosis of CSF leak to be made. CSF otorrhoea can initially be managed conservatively with bed rest and head elevation, but if not resolving may require lumbar drain, exploratory surgery and repair following discussion with lateral skull base surgeons.

94. Answer D

Temporary threshold shift (TTS) is a temporary sensorineural hearing loss (SNHL) that typically resolves within 24 hours. Permanent threshold shift (PTS) is a permanent hearing loss from noise exposure that does not improve with time. It is the outer (not inner) hair cells that are the most susceptible to noise-induced damage, with oxygen radical formation hypothesised as the cause with membranous and cellular damage. The stapedial reflex cannot reliably protect the cochlea from all sounds due to its latency of 10 ms, with a potential for unexpectedly loud sounds to thereby circumvent this. There is a higher likelihood of damage with exposure to higher intensities of sound (larger dB), prolonged exposure, as well as higher frequencies. Option D is therefore the most accurate statement.

95. Answer C

Option C is the correct answer. Superior semicircular canal dehiscence syndrome (SSCDS) was first described by Lloyd Minor in 1998. The vertigo with organ playing reported here (Tullio phenomenon) represents a third window phenomenon. This arises due to the formation of a third opening, the bony defect, between the superior semi-circular canal and the middle cranial fossa (the other openings to the inner ear are the oval and round windows). Patients may also report autophony, pulsatile tinnitus, hyperacusis, hearing loss and a sensation of "brain fog". An association often quoted in exam questions on SSCDS features wind instrument players, such as the saxophon-ist in this scenario. Otosclerosis could be possible given the strong family history, but autophony and sound-induced vertigo are more suggestive of a third window. Autophony is the only symptom that could favour patulous Eustachian tube, but Tullio's phenomenon is not part of this condition. There is an overlap with Meniere's disease; however, the autophony reported here is not frequently observed, nor does it constitute any of the diagnostic criteria for Meniere's disease.

96. Answer C

The radiological investigation of choice would be a high-resolution CT temporal bone scan to identify the presumed diagnosis of superior semicircular canal dehiscence and delineate the extent of the bony defect of the superior semicircular canal. This would also help guide the approach to surgery: transmastoid vs middle cranial fossa. Option D is incorrect however, since it only offers CT head rather than high-resolution CT temporal bones. In SSCDS, the investigation of choice would be cVEMP, which should demon-strate lower thresholds and increased amplitude compared to the normal side (making Option C correct). In SSCDS, the PTA is described as showing "supranormal thresholds", but this is not diagnostic in isolation. It could, however, be useful in counselling the patient with regards to post-operative hearing loss: semicircular canal plugging is asso-ciated with higher risk of total hearing loss compared to resurfacing alone. Stapedial reflexes should be present in SSCDS, but are often absent in otosclerosis: again this is not diagnostic, in isolation, for SSCDS. Tympanometry results alone would not confirm or refute a diagnosis of SSCDS.

97. Answer D

In this scenario, the symptoms are suggestive of vestibular migraine. Some triggers of vestibular migraine include dietary factors, stress or anxiety, alcohol, lack of sleep or poor hydration. Loud sound or abrupt head movements can aggravate symptoms during a migrainous episode but are not known triggers between episodes and should raise suspicion of a different diagnosis (e.g. BPPV/SSCD syndrome).

98. Answer B

In this scenario, the patient's episodic dizziness, headache, photophobia and phono-phobia suggest a diagnosis of vestibular migraine. The absence of a sustained hearing loss is helpful in differentiating vestibular migraine from Meniere's disease in which low-frequency unilateral hearing loss may be detected. A transitory low frequency hearing loss may been noted during a vestibular migraine attack. Increased time constants may be seen on rotation testing. Vestibular evoked myogenic potential (VEMP) abnor-malities are non-specific and variable.

99. Answer B

Cervical VEMPs (cVEMPs) measure sternocleidomastoid muscle responses triggered by sound stimuli and reflect saccular and inferior vestibular nerve function.

CHAPTER 2: HEAD AND NECK

1. A 28-year-old man is referred to your clinic because of changes to his voice. He tells you that people have always found it difficult to hear him, his voice gets hoarse, and he can be mistaken as female on the telephone due to vocal pitch changes. You find the following on flexible nasal endoscopy (Figure 2.1). Which of these is the most likely diagnosis?

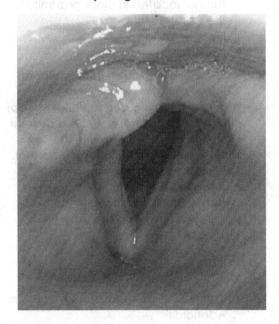

Figure 2.1 Vocal cord photo.

   A Spasmodic dysphonia
   B Sulcus vocalis
   C Vocal cord nodules
   D Sulcus vergeture
   E Reinke's oedema

2. Your patient is discussed in the local Head and Neck cancer multidisciplinary team (MDT) meeting for a T1bN0M0 glottic squamous cell carcinoma (SCC). Which of the following management plans is most likely to be suggested?
   A Surgery and post-operative radiotherapy
   B Chemotherapy
   C Radiotherapy
   D Chemotherapy and radiotherapy combined
   E Primary surgery with neck dissection

3. A 72-year-old patient presents to your clinic with a chronic history of regurgitation of undigested food, a sensation of a lump in the throat and intermittent coughing during meals. On further questioning, the patient also mentions a recent unintentional weight loss and change in voice. You suspect a pharyngeal pouch and plan to proceed with further investigations. Which of the following is NOT a common symptom or sign associated with a pharyngeal pouch?
   A Regurgitation of undigested food
   B Dysphagia
   C Halitosis
   D Aspiration pneumonia
   E Odynophagia

4. An 18-year-old student who sings in the college choir has been referred by her GP with a three-month history of a hoarse voice. It has worsened recently

DOI: 10.1201/9781003455059-2

during rehearsals for an upcoming performance and she is very anxious. What is the most likely diagnosis?

A Laryngeal papillomatosis
B Vocal cord palsy
C Vocal cord granuloma
D Vocal cord nodules
E Squamous cell carcinoma

5. Patients with head and neck squamous cell carcinoma (SCC) may be treated with intensity modulated radiation therapy (IMRT). Which of the following statements is TRUE regarding IMRT?

A IMRT is less precise in dose delivery compared to conventional radiotherapy.
B IMRT uses computer-controlled linear accelerators for precise radiation delivery.
C IMRT increases the radiation dose to surrounding normal critical structures.
D IMRT is a form of particle therapy.
E IMRT primarily increases the risk of side effects compared with conventional radiotherapy techniques.

6. A 47-year-old female patient presents to your clinic with a 12-year history of persistent oral lichen planus (OLP). Despite various topical treatments, her symptoms have fluctuated but never completely resolved. The lesions are predominantly reticular with some erosive areas. On examination, white reticular patches alongside areas of erythema and ulceration are noted bilaterally on the buccal mucosa and lateral borders of the tongue. Given the chronicity of her condition, she expresses concern regarding the potential for malignant transformation and seeks advice regarding long-term monitoring and any necessary interventions to mitigate this risk. What is the percentage risk of malignant transformation if present for over ten years?

A Less than 1%
B 2–5%

C 6–10%
D 11–15%
E Over 15%

7. A 62-year-old gardener presents with a lesion on the upper part of his right pinna. It has started bleeding on contact and become crusty and itchy and occasionally painful. On examination it is ulcerative, crusted and heaped at the edges. He proceeds to have a wide local excision with histopathology revealing squamous cell carcinoma (SCC). He returns to clinic 6 months later with a palpable ipsilateral parotid mass. Which of the following is not a risk factor for parotid metastasis from a cutaneous SCC?

A Primary tumour size >2 cm
B Incomplete excision margin
C Tumour located in close proximity to the parotid gland
D Desmoplastic lesion
E Lack of perineural invasion

8. A 32-year-old woman from southern China is being reviewed in the ENT emergency clinic due to unilateral epistaxis which has not improved despite topical Naseptin therapy in the community. Anterior rhinoscopy is normal. On flexible nasal endoscopy your colleague informs you they can see a friable area of mucosa in the postnasal space. What is the most likely diagnosis?

A Benign ulcer
B Rhinitis
C Non-keratinising carcinoma
D Keratinising squamous cell carcinoma
E Adenoiditis

9. A 32-year-old lady with biopsy-confirmed nasopharyngeal carcinoma is being discussed in your local head and neck cancer MDT. The tumour involves the nasopharynx with radiological evidence of extension into the parapharyngeal space, and there is no radiological evidence

of neck lymphadenopathy or metastatic deposits. What is the likely TNM
Staging?

A T2N0M0
B T1N0M0
C T1N1M0
D T3N0M0
E T2N1M0

10. A 24-year-old student from Bolivia is
referred to your clinic because of concerns
with appearance of her tongue (shown in
Figure 2.2). She has previously been diagnosed with Bell's palsy three times and has
been treated with oral steroids in the past.

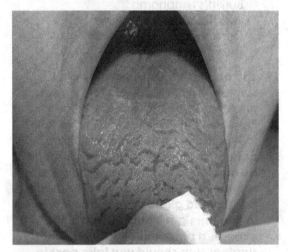

Figure 2.2 Tongue photo.

What is the most likely diagnosis?

A Syphilis
B Melkersson-Rosenthal syndrome
C Lyme Disease
D Guillain-Barré syndrome
E Maffucci syndrome

11. A 57-year-old professional actor is
diagnosed with T1aN0M0 laryngeal
cancer that appears exophytic and
encompasses the whole left vocal
cord. You are discussing management
options with the patient. Of the following, which is the most appropriate?

A Perform a European Laryngological
Society Classification (ELS) Type
I cordectomy

B Perform an ELS Classification Type II
cordectomy
C Perform an ELS Classification Type III
cordectomy
D Perform an ELS Classification Type IV
cordectomy
E Reconsider your plan and offer
radiotherapy

12. A 37-year-old man attends the emergency department four hours after
being assaulted in the street, sustaining
multiple punches to the face and neck.
His voice has progressively become
hoarse and he has some noisy breathing. What is the most likely finding on
flexible nasal endoscopy?

A Left vocal cord paralysis
B Pooling of saliva in the piriform fossa
C Laterally displaced larynx
D Glottic and supraglottic oedema with
mucosal haemorrhage
E Tongue base haematoma

13. A 37-year-old man attends the emergency department four hours after
being assaulted in the street, sustaining
multiple punches to the face and neck.
His voice has progressively become
hoarse and he has some noisy breathing. What is the name of the classification system used to best describe the
severity of laryngeal injury?

A Schaefer classification
B Schilder classification
C Sandifer classification
D Schamberg classification
E Shamblin classification

14. You are called urgently to the emergency department to review a 24-year-
old woman with shortness of breath
and intermittent stridor. Her oxygen
saturations are 98% on 1 L of oxygen.
She tells you that she has had similar events in the past. Her symptoms
have not improved with nebulised
adrenaline. She has a history of asthma
in childhood but is not currently taking any medication. The rest of her

observations and examination are normal. What is the most likely diagnosis?

A Laryngospasm

B Paradoxical vocal cord dysfunction

C Asthma

D Vocal cord nodules

E Bronchospasm

15. An 82-year-old woman is being seen in the emergency ENT clinic for otalgia. She reports a 2-month history of worsening left ear pain that spreads to her temporal region, pain on mastication, scalp tenderness and intermittent diplopia. Examination of her ear is normal. Recent blood tests organised by her GP are normal except for a raised erythrocyte sedimentation rate (ESR). What is the most likely clinical diagnosis?

A Necrotising otitis externa

B Herpes Zoster infection

C Trigeminal neuralgia

D Migraine

E Temporal arteritis (giant cell arteritis)

16. A 37-year-old lady with unilateral facial pain and headache is referred to you from her GP because of atypical features. The pain is sharp and shooting, localised to the malar region of the face and is reproducible on touch. She notices that it is worse on exposure to wind or when she brushes her teeth. What is the most likely clinical diagnosis?

A Sinusitis

B Herpes Zoster infection

C Trigeminal neuralgia

D Migraine

E Temporal arteritis (giant cell arteritis)

17. A 42-year-old lady attended your clinic due to worsening dysphonia, noisy breathing and shortness of breath on exertion. You perform a panendoscopy in theatre and find an abnormality at the level of the supraglottis. Of the following, which condition is the most likely cause of this abnormality?

A Amyloidosis

B Sarcoidosis

C Granulomatosis with polyangiitis

D Tuberculosis

E Rheumatoid arthritis

18. A 37-year-old lady who presented to your clinic with left-sided hearing loss and unilateral epistaxis was found to have a post-nasal space mass. You performed a biopsy and relevant imaging confirming nasopharyngeal carcinoma. The Epstein-Barr virus (EBV) status is positive from the histopathology. EBV is known to be associated with the following conditions, except for:

A T-Cell lymphoma

B Burkitt's lymphoma

C Infectious mononucleosis

D Nasopharyngeal carcinoma

E Hairy cell leukaemia

19. You are undertaking parathyroid surgery on a 52-year-old female who presented with hypercalcaemia. Preoperative investigations have failed to localise the adenoma and the patient undergoes a neck exploration. Having found normal-appearing left superior and inferior and right superior parathyroid glands you are now unable to find the right inferior gland in the expected anatomical position. What surgical step should you take next to localise the gland?

A Perform left hemithyroidectomy

B Open the left carotid sheath

C Perform total thyroidectomy

D Explore the retro-oesophageal area

E Explore the thymus

20. A 46-year-old lady with primary hyperparathyroidism is suspected to have a superior parathyroid adenoma, which is to be explored and excised for histopathology and symptomatic improvement. Which branchial pouch is responsible for the development of the superior parathyroid glands?

A First

B Second

C Third

D Fourth
E Fifth

21. **A 61-year-old man of West African origin is referred to your clinic by his GP with progressive neck swelling over the past 20 years. He has no symptoms of thyroid disease and does not have any concerns with voice, swallow or pain/pressure in the neck. What is the most likely cause of the neck swelling?**
    A Papillary thyroid carcinoma
    B Follicular thyroid carcinoma
    C Multinodular thyroid goitre
    D Follicular thyroid adenoma
    E Hashimoto's disease

22. **The embryological development of the tongue is from paired pharyngeal arches. Which arches are responsible for the normal anatomical development of the tongue?**
    A 1–4
    B 2–5
    C 3–6
    D 1–3
    E 2–4

23. **A 33-year-old woman presents to hospital with unprovoked acute tongue and lip swelling causing difficulty breathing and swallowing. She tells you this has happened twice in the past, but it had resolved without medical attention. She has no other medical history and takes no regular medication. What is the most useful diagnostic blood test to help you determine the diagnosis?**
    A Mast cell tryptase
    B Eosinophil count
    C C1 esterase inhibitor level
    D ESR
    E Serum angiotensin converting enzyme (ACE)

24. **You are performing a bicoronal osteoplastic flap as part of a joint craniofacial case with your maxillofacial colleagues,** this structure becomes visible as the flap is more superiorly raised and the junior doctors who are assisting ask you about it as a landmark. You inform them that this is the intersection of the coronal and sagittal suture lines and it is the point where the frontal bone and two parietal bones meet. What is the name of this bony landmark?
    A Inion
    B Rhinion
    C Bregma
    D Pterion
    E Asterion

25. **You are the on-call consultant who is asked to attend a major trauma call for a 20-year-old male poly-trauma patient who has sustained multiple craniofacial injuries and may need a front-of-neck airway. The trauma team lead and neurosurgeon feel that the most significant injury is to the lateral side of the head and this injury predisposes him to an epidural hematoma. Which bones constitute this anatomical weak spot?**
    A Frontal—Parietal—Sphenoid—Occipital
    B Frontal—Parietal—Temporal—Sphenoid
    C Frontal—Sphenoid—Occipital—Zygomatic
    D Frontal—Sphenoid—Zygomatic—Clivus
    E Frontal—Temporal—Occipital—Parietal

26. **A 35-year-old woman presents to the ENT clinic with a recent history of facial weakness on the right side. Clinical examination reveals a lower motor neuron type facial nerve palsy. Which of the following nerves is not a branch of the facial nerve?**
    A Chorda tympani
    B Temporal
    C Nerve to stapedius
    D Lesser petrosal
    E Posterior auricular

27. A 52-year-old woman presents to your clinic with a history of progressive difficulty in swallowing solid foods over the last year. She mentions that she often has to drink water to help get the food down and has noticed regurgitation of undigested food. Recently, she has also been experiencing chest pain and has lost a significant amount of weight due to these symptoms. With these symptoms, you suspect oesophageal achalasia. What is the underlying pathological mechanism of this condition?

A Severe gastro-oesophageal reflux leading to Schatzki ring

B Significant peristalsis in the oesophagus

C Lower oesophageal sphincter insufficiency causing reduced pressure in the lower oesophagus

D Loss of ganglion cells in the myenteric plexus

E *Trypanosoma brucei* infection

28. A 45-year-old man presents to your clinic for his six-week post-operative follow-up after undergoing a right neck dissection to manage metastatic squamous cell carcinoma of the head and neck region. He has recovered well from the procedure; however, he mentions a new onset of difficulty in shoulder movement and a noticeable winging of his scapula on the operated side, particularly when he pushes against resistance or tries to lift his arm above shoulder level. On examination, you notice a prominent winging of his right scapula as he attempts to push against the wall. You suspect nerve damage and now need to identify which cervical nerve roots were likely affected during the surgery to provide an accurate diagnosis and management plan. Which cervical nerve roots are most likely to have been damaged during the neck dissection?

A C5
B C6
C C7
D C5–6
E C5–7

29. A 45-year-old male undergoes a submandibular gland excision due to recurrent sialadenitis. Post-operatively, he complains of numbness and altered sensation on the anterior two thirds of the tongue on the side of the surgery. Upon further evaluation, you also find a loss of taste sensation. Which nerve is most likely to have been injured during the submandibular gland excision, given the patient's post-operative symptoms?

A Hypoglossal nerve
B Glossopharyngeal nerve
C Lingual nerve
D Inferior alveolar nerve
E Vagus nerve

30. A 62-year-old female undergoes a right hemithyroidectomy for a Thy3f nodule. What is the risk of malignancy on histopathological analysis of this nodule?

A 5%
B 10%
C 30%
D 45%
E 50%

31. A 61-year-old female with no significant comorbidities is on your elective operating list for a right hemithyroidectomy for a 2 cm Thy3f lesion. The procedure is performed by your registrar and there are no immediate post-operative concerns. When you see her in the clinic for follow-up, she has noticed that the pitch of her voice when singing in church has changed and she can no longer reach the higher notes, although her conversational voice is normal. The scar has healed nicely and there is no obvious asymmetry of the vocal cords on flexible nasal endoscopy. Which muscle is innervated by the nerve likely to have been injured during the operation?

A Vocalis
B Cricothyroid
C Posterior crico-arytenoid
D Oblique arytenoid
E Transverse arytenoid

32. **You are reviewing a 36-year-old female in the pre-operative area who has been listed for a completion thyroidectomy following a previous left hemithyroidectomy for a 4 cm follicular carcinoma 4 months ago. The pathology report indicates the tumour has been completely excised. This is the first time you have met the patient since she had been assessed and listed by a colleague. You notice her voice is weak and therefore perform flexible nasendoscopy, noting a paralysed left vocal cord. You discuss with a colleague who suggests using intra-operative nerve monitoring for the case which he has recently started using, but you are yet to trial. Of the following, which is the most appropriate?**
A Perform completion thyroidectomy using intra-operative nerve monitoring
B Perform completion thyroidectomy using your standard operative approach
C Perform completion thyroidectomy with a covering tracheostomy
D Cancel the case and plan rediscussion at the thyroid MDT
E Cancel the case and book a follow-up ultrasound for 1 month

33. **A 64-year-old male with hypertension and mitral stenosis presents with a weak voice and a left vocal cord palsy. What is the most likely cardiac cause of his symptoms?**
A Left atrial enlargement
B Pseudoaneurysm
C Pulmonary artery hypertension
D Atrial myxoma
E Left apical cardiomyopathy

34. **A 52-year-old man presents to your clinic with recurrent neck swelling and pain during meals. The swelling is becoming increasingly frequent, although he has never had an acute infection or abscess requiring drainage. Examination of his neck is normal. Given the symptoms, what is the best investigation to diagnose this condition?**
A Sialogram
B Ultrasound scan
C CT scan
D MRI scan
E X-ray

35. **A 52-year-old man presents to your clinic with 3 cm mass in the tail of his parotid gland. You plan to perform a superficial parotidectomy and are undertaking informed consent. You mention the risk of nerve damage and facial weakness. The patient asks about other nerves in the parotid gland that could be at risk during the surgery as he is worried about having a dry mouth. The following nerve is responsible for secretomotor function to the parotid gland:**
A Trigeminal nerve
B Chorda tympani
C Lingual nerve
D Glossopharyngeal nerve
E Hypoglossal

36. **A 47-year-old female presents to your head and neck clinic with bilateral parotid swelling. On review of her medical records you note she has hypertension, previous transient ischaemic attacks, is a current smoker and her HBA1c = 7%. Her sister and brother have rheumatoid arthritis. There are no red flag symptoms and on examination both glands are diffusely swollen and non-tender and there are no skin changes. What is the most likely cause of the parotid swelling?**
A Sjogren's syndrome
B Diabetes
C Pleomorphic adenoma
D Mumps
E Lymphoma

37. A 42-year-old heavy goods vehicle driver has been referred to you due to worsening snoring over the past year with considerable daytime sleepiness. On examination he has grade 3 tonsils and is Mallampati grade 1. You note a deviated nasal septum with reduced airflow through the left side of the nose. You arrange a sleep study that suggests moderate to severe sleep apnoea. Of the following, which is the most appropriate first-line management?
   A List for septoplasty
   B Mandibular advancement splint
   C Tonsillectomy and uvulectomy/ uvuloplasty
   D Continuous positive airway pressure device (CPAP)
   E Nasal oxygen cannula

38. A 69-year-old man with a high BMI and excessive snoring and daytime sleepiness has a sleep study showing moderate obstructive sleep apnoea. He is started on a continuous positive airway pressure device (CPAP) however is unable to tolerate it. Examination reveals a Mallampati III airway with oropharyngeal crowding. You undertake a detailed cephalometric and anatomical assessment to guide your decision making regarding the success of surgery. Which of the following features also increases the risk of obstructive sleep apnoea (OSA)?
   A Mandibular or maxillary deficiency
   B Short palatoglossal arch
   C Superior position of the hyoid
   D Reduced sagittal projection of the face
   E Prominent lingual frenulum

39. Which of the following is not an indication for PET-CT in the diagnostic work-up and staging of head and neck cancer:
   A p16 positive head and neck SCC of unknown primary
   B T4 nasopharyngeal carcinoma
   C T4 supraglottic laryngeal SCC
   D T4 hypopharyngeal SCC
   E p16 negative head and neck SCC of unknown primary

40. A 41-year-old man attends your clinic with a parotid gland swelling. On examination, you palpate a mass within the gland, yet there is no evidence of head and neck lymphadenopathy and the rest of the ENT examination is normal. An initial ultrasound reveals a localised parotid mass but cannot delineate whether it extends into the deep lobe of the parotid or not. Which imaging modality will best demonstrate whether this lesion has deep lobe extension or not?
   A CT scan with contrast imaging
   B MRI scan with gadolinium based contrast
   C MRI scan with non-echo planar diffusion weighted imaging
   D MRI scan with diffusion weighted imaging
   E MRI scan with short tau inversion recovery imaging

41. A 44-year-old lady is referred to your head and neck clinic with a slow-growing right-sided angle of jaw swelling. It is not painful nor has it ever been infected. The swelling is a cosmetic concern for her and does not change with eating or swallowing. Other than this 3 cm, soft, non-fixed lump, the ENT examination is normal. An ultrasound scan with fine needle aspiration is organised, and cytology suggests a likely pleomorphic adenoma. What percentage of pleomorphic adenomas are found in the parotid gland?
   A 5%
   B 10%
   C 25%
   D 50%
   E 75%

42. What is the percentage likelihood of malignant change of a pleomorphic adenoma in the first five years?
    A 1.5%
    B 2.5%
    C 5%
    D 10%
    E 20%

43. A 30-year-old female presents with a growing thyroid nodule. An ultrasound is undertaken confirming a 5 cm U5 nodule and two ipsilateral 2 cm cervical nodes. Fine needle aspiration is consistent with papillary cell carcinoma. What is the next most appropriate investigation?
    A CT neck and chest with contrast
    B CT neck and chest without contrast
    C MRI neck and chest with contrast
    D Radioactive iodine uptake test
    E PET-CT

44. An 46 year old female has been referred to your clinic with a parotid swelling and a facial nerve palsy. The lesion is painful and has been slowly growing over the past year. He is a current smoker. Concerned about a potential parotid gland malignancy, you send him for an ultrasound scan with tissue sampling and staging scans. What is the most likely diagnosis?
    A Lymphoma
    B Acinic cell carcinoma
    C Mucoepidermoid carcinoma
    D Squamous cell carcinoma
    E Adenoid cystic carcinoma

45. A 67-year-old man, initially referred due to a new tonsil mass, has undergone staging scans and biopsy, which confirmed squamous cell carcinoma. During the head and neck cancer MDT discussion, the histopathologist reports an HPV/P16 positive biopsy sample. Which strain of HPV is most likely to cause oropharyngeal SCC?
    A 6
    B 11
    C 16
    D 18
    E All of the above are equally common

46. Which anatomical sub-site of the oropharynx is most likely to develop HPV/P16 positive squamous cell carcinoma?
    A Buccal mucosa
    B Tongue
    C Tonsil
    D Tongue base
    E Piriform fossa

47. A 57-year-old farmer consults you in your head and neck clinic about an irritating dome-shaped scaly lump under the angle of the mandible, which grew rapidly initially but fluctuates in size. What is the most likely diagnosis of this lesion?
    A Squamous cell carcinoma
    B Basal cell carcinoma
    C Pyogenic granuloma
    D Keratoacanthoma
    E Sebaceous cyst

48. What nerves are responsible for the function of the pharyngeal phase of swallowing?
    A Trigeminal and glossopharyngeal
    B Glossopharyngeal and vagus
    C Trigeminal and vagus
    D Facial and glossopharyngeal
    E Trigeminal and facial

49. A 61-year-old lady with a history of hypertension presents with new-onset persistent hoarseness. Following a thorough ENT examination and imaging studies, a localised lesion on the left vocal fold is identified, with histology confirming squamous cell carcinoma (SCC). No lymphadenopathy or distant metastasis is observed. What would affect the final staging of this lesion?
    A Extension onto the underside of the vocal fold
    B Extension onto the vocal process

C Extension onto the false vocal fold

D Extension up to the anterior commissure

E Depth of invasion of more than 5 mm

50. **An 81-year-old man is referred to you with progressively worsening difficulties in swallowing. He experiences regurgitation of food frequently during meals, making it almost impossible to finish a meal. He has recently recovered from a chest infection. Upon neck examination, you palpate a soft, compressible mass in the left side of his neck behind the sternocleidomastoid. Auscultation of the mass reveals gurgling sounds. What is the name of this auscultatory sign?**

A Boyce's

B Grisel's

C Tullio's

D Aquino's

E Brown's

51. **A 37-year-old professional trombone player is referred to you due to persistent throat irritation, frequent need to clear the throat and intermittent changes in voice quality accompanied by throat congestion. ENT examination and flexible nasal endoscopy reveal no abnormalities. There is no evidence of head and neck lymphadenopathy or palpable masses. What is the most likely diagnosis?**

A Pharyngeal pouch

B Laryngopharyngeal reflux

C Laryngocele

D Reinke's oedema

E Chronic laryngitis

52. **A 72-year-old man with confirmed hypopharyngeal SCC on histology comes to see you in clinic for follow-up and to receive the diagnosis and update from your MDT meeting. Where is the most likely anatomical location within the hypopharynx that an SCC arises from?**

A Vocal cord

B Cricoid cartilage

C Piriform fossa

D Post cricoid

E Posterior pharyngeal wall

53. **A 37-year-old lady comes to see you with left pulsatile tinnitus which has not improved with meditation or using tinnitus therapy guidance/websites. Her audiogram is normal but she has a slightly lower amplitude, type A tympanogram. On examination there is a red mass medial to the inferior aspect of the pars tensa. What blood vessel is most likely to predominantly supply this tumour?**

A Internal maxillary

B Facial

C Lingual

D Ascending pharyngeal

E Superior thyroid

54. **A 54-year-old male presented to your clinic with a growing parotid lump and normal facial function. Fine needle aspiration and imaging reveal a 15 mm adenoid cystic carcinoma in the superficial parotid gland with 2 ipsilateral neck nodes in level 2, the largest of which is 2.5 cm. Which of the following is the most appropriate management?**

A Total parotidectomy and neck dissection, with preservation of the facial nerve if uninvolved by disease at time of surgery and adjuvant radiotherapy

B Total parotidectomy and neck dissection, with sacrifice of the facial nerve and adjuvant radiotherapy

C Superficial parotidectomy and neck dissection, with preservation of the facial nerve if uninvolved by disease at time of surgery and adjuvant radiotherapy

D Primary radiotherapy

E Superficial parotidectomy and neck dissection, with preservation of the facial nerve if uninvolved by disease at time of surgery

55. **A 47-year-old male presents with left level 2 neck lump. Core biopsy is consistent with HPV positive SCC. You arrange an MRI neck and a PET-CT, that reveal a 3 cm level 2 neck node without**

radiological evidence of extra-nodal extension, but the primary site is not determined. You plan to perform a bilateral tonsillectomy and tongue base mucosectomy. With regards to the management of the neck disease which of the following is most appropriate?

A Neck dissection is not required since the diagnosis is likely to be made by the tongue base mucosectomy or tonsillectomy and the neck is best managed with radiotherapy

B Perform a selective neck dissection level 2–4

C Perform a supraomohyoid neck dissection

D Perform a selective neck dissection level 2–5

E Perform an excisional biopsy of the 3 cm level 2 neck node

56. A 31-year-old male undergoes an MRI neck for a growing left neck lump. The imaging shows a 4 cm cystic and necrotic node in left level 2 but no other evidence of a primary site. The rest of the head and neck examination, including flexible nasendoscopy, is normal. You request an ultrasound guided fine needle aspiration (FNA) which reveals HPV positive SCC. The patient tells you his brother has recently undergone treatment for tonsil cancer. What is the most appropriate next step in management?

A Fludeoxyglucose (18F) PET-CT

B CT neck

C DOTATATE PET

D Further imaging is not required and the neck lump should be excised

E Referral to genetics

57. A 51-year-old male is referred to you due to ongoing foreign body sensation in his throat associated with intermittent voice changes and pitch changes. He is a non-smoker who works as a publicist. Endoscopic examination in clinic reveals the lesion pictured in Figure 2.3. What is the likely diagnosis?

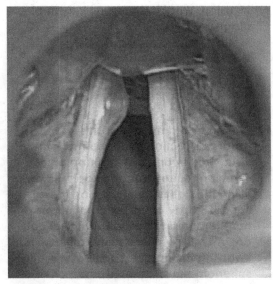

Figure 2.3 Throat photo.

A Squamous cell carcinoma

B Reinke's oedema

C Vocal cord cyst

D Vocal cord granuloma

E Vocal cord nodule

58. A 22-year-old man with recurrent tonsillitis is referred to your clinic by his GP for consideration of tonsillectomy. He has had 3 episodes of tonsillitis requiring antibiotics, each year for the past two years. Based on the SIGN/NICE (Scottish Intercollegiate Guidelines Network/National Institute for Health and Care Excellence) criteria, how many episodes as a minimum are required per annum for two years to be eligible for a tonsillectomy for recurrent tonsillitis?

A Two

B Three

C Four

D Five

E Seven

59. A 61-year-old lady is referred with a left neck mass. She has an ultrasound scan and fine needle aspirate revealing a Thy3f lesion. She undergoes a diagnostic hemithyroidectomy and shows evidence of blood vessel and capsular

invasion. What is the most likely final diagnosis?

A Anaplastic carcinoma
B Follicular carcinoma
C Follicular adenoma
D Medullary carcinoma
E Lymphoma

60. A 36-year-old male presents with nasal obstruction, reduced monocular visual acuity and ophthalmoplegia. Examination reveals an exophytic mass filling the right side of the post-nasal space. Biopsy of the lesion confirms a non-keratinising nasopharyngeal cancer. An MRI reveals an infiltrative lesion involving the right fossa of Rosenmuller, sphenoid sinus, ethmoid sinus, cavernous sinus and orbital apex. There are two 4 cm bilateral neck nodes. What is the most appropriate management strategy?

A Primary radiotherapy with concurrent platinum chemotherapy
B Primary radiotherapy with concurrent EGFR inhibitor
C Nasopharyngectomy with adjuvant radiotherapy
D Endoscopic nasopharyngectomy
E Palliation

61. A 35-year-old woman presents with recurrent hoarseness and has been diagnosed with recurrent respiratory papillomatosis (RRP). She enquires about preventative measures for her children. Which vaccine provides preventative cover for RRP?

A Gardasil
B Cervarix
C Aciclovir
D Valaciclovir
E Ganciclovir

62. A 68-year-old man had a total laryngopharyngectomy with gastric pull-up five days ago for laryngeal squamous cell carcinoma. He is now suffering from post-operative dehydration and has been diagnosed with acute tubular

necrosis. What electrolyte disturbance is most likely to be of concern on blood sampling?

A Hypercalcaemia
B Hypernatraemia
C Hyponatraemia
D Hyperkalaemia
E Hypokalaemia

63. You are on the ITU reviewing a 64-year-old obese man in decompensated liver failure due to alcohol abuse. Two weeks previously he had a percutaneous tracheostomy for ventilatory weaning. He remains sedated and ventilated. He now has profuse pulsatile bleeding from the tracheostomy stoma and through the tracheostomy tube. He is haemodynamically unstable. The ITU and resusciation team are already in attendance. What is the most appropriate course of action?

A CT angiogram
B Perform the Utley manoeuvre and inform emergency theatres that you need a theatre immediately
C Pack the tracheostomy stoma with Surgicel
D Attempt bedside electrocautery
E Remove the tracheostomy tube and attempt oral intubation

64. A 26-year-old woman presents with a persistent anterior neck lump following a severe upper respiratory tract infection. The lump was initially red and has been treated with antibiotics. Now, the skin appears normal, but a firm lump remains. On examination, there is a 3x4 cm lump in the anterior neck in the midline that moves on tongue protrusion. What is the most important pre-operative investigation?

A CT neck with contrast
B Thyroid function tests
C Ultrasound neck
D MRI neck
E Pure tone audiogram

65. A 57-year-old man presents with pressure symptoms in the neck and an enlarging neck mass. Ultrasound reveals a large multinodular goitre, with all nodules classified as U2. You decide to proceed with a total thyroidectomy. During the operation, while teaching about neck anatomy, you point out Joll's triangle. What nerve would you find in this region?
    A Recurrent laryngeal
    B Internal branch of superior laryngeal
    C External branch of superior laryngeal
    D Hypoglossal
    E Vagus

66. During a neck dissection, you are explaining the anatomy of the digastric muscle to your registrar. What nerve innervates the anterior belly of the digastric muscle?
    A Trigeminal
    B Facial
    C Glossopharyngeal
    D Vagus
    E Hypoglossal

67. You are seeing a 41-year-old woman in your clinic who presented with a thyroid nodule. She has undergone a diagnostic hemithyroidectomy on the basis of a pre-operative ultrasound-guided fine needle aspiration. The pathologist at the MDT meeting tells you that the surgical specimen contained numerous psammoma bodies and orphan Annie nuclei. What is the likely diagnosis?
    A Follicular thyroid carcinoma
    B Anaplastic thyroid carcinoma
    C Papillary thyroid carcinoma
    D Oncocytic thyroid carcinoma
    E Follicular adenoma

68. You are reviewing a 54-year-old male who has been on long-term CPAP for obstructive sleep apnoea. He reports he is having problems tolerating the device due to increased pressure requirements and a persistent mask leak. On examination you note a BMI of 45 kg/m², a deviated septum and bilateral turbinate hypertrophy, grade 3 tonsils and significant collapse on Muller manoeuvre. What is the most appropriate next step?
    A Referral for consideration of bariatric surgery
    B List for tonsillectomy
    C List for uvulopalatopharyngoplasty (UVPP)
    D Prescribe a course of topical nasal steroids
    E List for septoplasty

69. An 87-year-old man presents to your head and neck clinic with a history of progressive dysphagia, regurgitation, recurrent chest infections and weight loss. What is the best investigation to confirm this diagnosis?
    A Plain film X-ray
    B CT scan
    C MRI scan
    D Barium swallow
    E Panendoscopy and biopsy

70. A 50-year-old male undergoes a laryngopharyngectomy and free flap reconstruction for a locally advanced hypopharyngeal SCC. Of the following, which flap gives the best swallowing outcome?
    A Anterolateral thigh flap
    B Deltopectoral flap
    C Radial forearm free flap
    D Jejunal free flap
    E Gastric pull-up

71. A 37-year-old woman comes to your clinic six months after a superficial parotidectomy. She complains of gustatory sweating that affects her quality of life. You offer botulinum toxin A treatment. How is it administered?
    A Topically
    B Intradermally
    C Subcutaneous
    D Intraglandular
    E Intramuscular

72. **A 37-year-old woman is back in your clinic six months after a superficial parotidectomy. She experiences gustatory sweating but no facial nerve weakness. What is the underlying pathophysiology of her symptoms?**
    A Sympathetic parotid gland fibres connecting with parasympathetic sweat gland fibres in the skin, mediated by acetylcholine
    B Parasympathetic parotid gland fibres connecting with sympathetic sweat gland fibres in the skin, mediated by acetylcholine
    C Sympathetic parotid gland fibres connecting with sympathetic sweat gland fibres in the skin, mediated by acetylcholine
    D Parasympathetic parotid gland fibres connecting with parasympathetic sweat gland fibres in the skin, mediated by acetylcholine
    E None of the above

73. **A 32-year-old female presents to your neck lump clinic with a growing left-sided lateral neck lump. After thorough investigations, it turns out to be papillary thyroid cancer with regional lymph node metastasis. What is the most appropriate management plan?**
    A Neck dissection
    B Total thyroidectomy and neck dissection
    C Total thyroidectomy and neck dissection with radioactive iodine therapy
    D Radiotherapy
    E Radioactive iodine therapy alone

74. **A patient is admitted with a head injury and subsequent extradural haematoma. Which skull base foramen or fissure does the blood vessel most likely injured in this patient run through?**
    A Foramen lacerum
    B Foramen ovale
    C Foramen spinosum
    D Foramen rotundum
    E Petrotympanic fissure

75. **A 66-year-old mechanic with a long history of smoking presents with a hoarse voice and breathlessness. You notice a small pleural effusion on his chest X-ray. What is the most likely finding on nasendoscopy?**
    A Laryngeal SCC
    B Vocal cord nodules
    C Reinke's oedema
    D Vocal cord palsy
    E Laryngo-pharyngeal reflux

76. **What is the most appropriate first-line investigation for an adult with an unexplained vocal cord palsy?**
    A Plain chest X-ray
    B MRI brain
    C CT neck and thorax
    D Panendoscopy and biopsy
    E Referral to speech and language therapy

77. **A 27-year-old man presents with a persistent central tongue abnormality shown in Figure 2.4. He is a current smoker. What is the most appropriate management?**
    A Steroid-based mouthwash

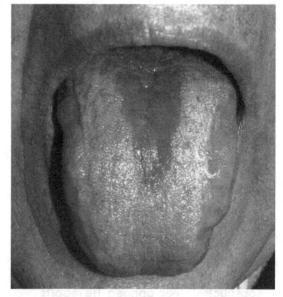

Figure 2.4 Tongue value.
By Klaus D. Peter, Wiehl, Germany—Own work, CC BY 3.0 de, https://commons.wikimedia.org/w/index.php?curid=22453275

B Antifungal capsules/tablets
C Antifungal lozenges
D Oral antibiotics
E Biopsy

78. **A 59-year-old male is being discussed at the head and neck MDT. After appropriate investigations he has been diagnosed with a T4aN1M0 supraglottic cancer with a non-mobile vocal cord. He has mild hypertension and is a smoker. Of the following, which is the most appropriate management?**
    A Total laryngectomy with bilateral neck dissection and post operative radiotherapy
    B Primary radiotherapy
    C Chemoradiotherapy
    D Supraglottic partial laryngectomy, bilateral neck dissections and post-operative radiotherapy
    E T4a supraglottic cancer is unresectable and the patient should be offered palliative radiotherapy

79. **A 49-year-old lady presents with a blistering rash and oral ulceration. Blood tests show antibodies to skin desmosome (desmoglein-3). What is the likely diagnosis?**
    A Pemphigoid
    B Pemphigus
    C Guttate psoriasis
    D Erythema multiforme
    E Aphthous ulceration

80. **A 54-year-old man has been referred from the respiratory team for consideration of surgical management of his obstructive sleep apnoea. His recent sleep study shows an apnoea-hypopnoea index (AHI) = 41 events/hour, with lowest desaturation of 79%. He has been unable to use CPAP due to claustrophobia. After assessment you feel he is an appropriate candidate for uvulopalatopharyngoplasty (UVPP). You are discussing the procedure and the chances of success in managing his**

OSA. **Of the following options which is most important in determining the success of UVPP?**
    A Friedman stage 1
    B Friedman stage 3
    C BMI over 40
    D Pre-operative elongated uvula
    E Pre-operative increased nasal resistance

81. **You are reviewing a 47-year-old male in clinic after uvulopalatopharyngoplasty for severe OSA (preoperative AHI = 36 events/hour, lowest desaturation 89%) having failed a CPAP trial. Initially he felt that his snoring was better but over the last few months he feels that he is snoring as loudly as before. You decide to repeat his sleep study which shows an AHI of 14 events/hour with the lowest desaturation of 94%. The patient is concerned he might need more surgery. Which statement is correct regarding the success of the first procedure?**
    A Successful sleep surgery is defined as a reduction in AHI by 50% and an AHI <20
    B The surgery has not been successful since the AHI >10
    C The success of sleep surgery cannot be defined in terms of the change in AHI
    D The surgery has not been successful because the lowest desaturation is <97%
    E The most common method to define success of sleep surgery is a composite measure of post-operative AHI and Epworth sleepiness score

82. **A 68-year-old lady who lives in a care home due to her dementia was suspected of choking on her lunch and now has absolute dysphagia. She has been brought to the emergency department, is unable to eat or drink, but is not complaining of any pain. She has normal observations and no evidence of surgical emphysema on neck examination. The oral examination is normal, and she cannot tolerate a flexible nasal**

endoscopy. What is the most appropriate initial investigation?

A Antero-posterior and lateral soft tissue neck plain radiograph
B MRI neck with contrast
C Erect chest X-ray
D Barium swallow
E Panendoscopy

83. A 47-year-old florist attends your clinic due to persistent left-sided throat discomfort and soreness. She has experienced weight loss and has a 2.5 cm left tonsil mass and a mass in her left neck on examination. Biopsy confirms squamous cell carcinoma (P16 negative) and CT neck and chest identifies an ipsilateral 6.5 cm node, and no lung metastases. What is the most likely MDT staging for this tumour?

A T1N1M0
B T2N1M0
C T2N2M0
D T2N3M0
E T3N2M0

84. You are considering a surgical approach to address a patient's dysphagia and are reviewing the relevant anatomy. Which cranial nerve innervates the stylopharyngeus muscle?

A Facial nerve
B Glossopharyngeal
C Vagus
D Spinal accessory
E Hypoglossal

85. A 89-year-old lady presents with diarrhoea and develops bilateral parotid gland swelling. What is the most helpful initial blood test?

A C-reactive protein
B Erythrocyte sedimentation rate
C Full blood count
D Renal function test
E Liver function test

86. A 47-year-old barber presents with a lesion on the tongue that needs laser resection. Which laser is best used for this resection?

A KTP
B CO2
C Argon
D Nd:YAG
E Ruby

87. During a joint voice clinic, you notice a patient has phonation associated with jitter. What does jitter in voice pathology represent?

A Changes in amplitude
B Changes in voice resonance
C Perturbation of pitch period
D Voice power
E Phonation frequency

88. A 27-year-old male recently diagnosed with HIV is referred to the head and neck clinic. What is the most common presentation of HIV to the head and neck clinic?

A Parotid cyst/lumps
B Oral candidiasis
C Adenotonsillar hypertrophy
D Neck lump
E Necrotising otitis externa

89. A 62-year-old painter who has been a smoker presents with a faint raspy voice and faint white lesions on both sides of the vocal cords. Although he is worried about the risks of general anaesthesia, he agrees for you to undertake a biopsy in theatre which reveals severe dysplasia. When you see the patient for follow-up, he asks about his future risk of laryngeal cancer if he has no further treatment.

A <5%
B No risk
C 20%
D 30%
E 75%

90. A patient you are seeing in your thyroid clinic has medullary thyroid cancer, which turns out to be a germline genetic mutation in the *RET* gene, diagnosed by the clinical genetics team as MEN2A. Her daughter is 3 years old and

is being tested for the mutation. If she has inherited the mutation, when would thyroidectomy usually be indicated/advised?

A By 6 months old
B By 5 years old
C By 10 years old
D As soon as possible
E Once 16 years old

91. A 23-year-old presents with a sudden-onset sore throat and grey-white coating over his tonsils which extends down his pharynx and is very adherent when swabbed. He cannot eat and drink. There is no airway compromise, he is septic, has been spiking temperatures and has significant bilateral lymphadenopathy. He works with refugees. What is the best next step in his management?

A Admit for intravenous fluids, benzyl-penicillin and send a Paul Bunnell test
B Broad spectrum antibiotics and CT neck with contrast
C Intravenous azithromycin and anti-toxin infusion, after discussion with microbiology
D Oral penicillin V and send home, with safety netting advice
E Call ITU for immediate assessment, start IV antibiotics

92. An 89-year-old patient presents with a chicken food bolus which she is adamant has no bone in it. However, she can still feel something present in her throat and is drinking but not eating well. She has hypertension, a previous myocardial infarction and chronic obstructive pulmonary disease (COPD) and is on anti-platelet medications. The plain radiograph is suspicious for a bony foreign body, but not definitive. Which is the most appropriate next step?

A Rigid oesophagoscopy and removal of foreign body
B Admit and review in the morning

C CT neck with contrast
D Oesophagogastroduodenoscopy (OGD)
E CT neck without contrast

93. A 91-year-old patient with diagnosed high-grade lymphoma is shown to have upper tracheal compression on a staging CT from her mediastinal disease. She has not yet had radiotherapy, but has started some palliative chemotherapy. On review she has some shortness of breath on exertion, but is not in respiratory distress and has no active stridor. The haematologists are concerned about her airway. You work with them, the patient and their family to form a plan. What would be the best next step?

A Awake fibreoptic intubation
B Awake local anaesthetic tracheostomy
C Routine intubation and tracheostomy under general anaesthetic
D Trial of steroids and close observation
E Urgent radiotherapy

94. A 67-year-old patient is having a laryngopharyngectomy and free-flap reconstruction. Their past medical history includes a colorectal cancer resection, hypertension and they had a radiologically inserted gastrostomy (RIG) before starting treatment. Their Allen test is abnormal bilaterally. What is the best reconstructive option for them?

A Radial forearm free flap (RFFF)
B Anterolateral thigh flap (ALT)
C Scapula free flap
D Gastric pull-up
E Jejunal free flap

95. Which of the following statements regarding depth of invasion in oral cavity cancer is true?

A Depth of invasion can be defined as the vertical distance between the most superficial and the deepest parts of the tumour

B Depth of invasion is not a good predictor of lymph node metastasis

C Depth of invasion greater than 15
mm increases the TNM T stage to T4

D Depth of invasion can be defined as
the vertical distance between basement membrane and deepest part
of the tumour

E Depth of invasion greater than 20
mm is an indication for post-operative chemotherapy

96. **You see a 25-year-old woman in clinic
with a new diagnosis of papillary thyroid carcinoma. She tells you she has
several first-degree relatives who have
undergone bowel surgery. Which of the
following is the most likely diagnosis?**
A Hirschsprung disease
B Pendred syndrome
C Cowden syndrome
D Familial adenomatous polyposis
E DICER 1 syndrome

97. **A 19-year-old man attends clinic with
a thyroid nodule and tells you he has
recently been diagnosed with corneal
nerve thickening. What syndrome
is most likely to cause both of these
conditions?**
A MEN2B
B MEN2A
C MEN1
D Werner syndrome
E Carney complex type 1

98. **Which of the following is not recognised
as a risk factor for parastomal recur-
rence following total laryngectomy for
SCC?**
A Advanced T stage
B Subglottic tumour location
C Pre-operative tracheostomy
D Central compartment nodal
metastases
E Free-flap pharyngeal reconstruction

99. **A 40-year-old female attends the
two-week-wait clinic with painful
lace-like white lesions on her left buccal mucosa. What is the most appropriate first line management?**

A Antiseptic mouthwash
B Topical steroid
C CO2 laser excision
D Methotrexate
E Propranolol

100. **You note milky fluid in the drain on
day 2 following a left selective neck
dissection. What is the most appropri-
ate first course of action?**
A Octreotide 200 mcg TDS
B Long chain fatty acid diet
C Nasogastric tube feeding
D Nurse head down
E Medium chain fatty acid diet

101. **A 19-year-old man is brought into
the emergency department with a
knife protruding from the left neck
anterior to the mid-point of sternocleidomastoid. He is haemodynamically stable and there is no active
bleeding or expanding haematoma.
Which of the following is the most
appropriate initial management
following primary and secondary
surveys?**
A Remove the knife and probe the
wound with a culture swab
B Move the patient to theatre for intubation and surgical exploration
C Call the vascular surgery team
D Arrange a CT angiogram of the
head and neck
E Administer a dose of tranexamic acid

102. **You request a CT in the pre-operative
work-up of a patient with a large
multinodular thyroid goitre, and the
radiologist comments on an aberrant
right subclavian artery. Which of the
following will you be likely to encounter intra-operatively?**
A High innominate artery
B Retro-oesophageal right inferior
parathyroid gland
C Non-recurrent right recurrent laryngeal nerve
D Extra-laryngeal bifurcation of the
right recurrent laryngeal nerve
E Duplication of the superior thyroid
artery

ANSWERS

Head and Neck

1. **Answer D**

   A sulcus is an invagination on the surface of the vocal fold resulting from a thin-ning of the superficial lamina propria. Sulcus vergeture refers to a sulcus that spans the length of a vocal fold. The picture shows a left sulcus vergeture (the right side is incompletely seen). Patients usually report lifelong hoarseness, suggesting it is potentially a developmental disorder. Sulcus vergeture causes complex vocal dysfunction. The voice is typically harsh and reedy with vocal strain and feminisa-tion. In contrast, sulcus vocalis occurs in a limited area of a vocal fold within areas of adjacent inflammation. The vocal symptoms of sulcus vocalis tend to be inter-mittent. Treatment options for sulcus include phonosurgery, specifically vocal cord augmentation or injection, and speech therapy, mainly aimed at strengthening the voice.

2. **Answer C**

   This patient has an early stage (Stage I) glottic SCC. T1b tumours involve both true vocal folds. Primary radiotherapy is an effective treatment for early-stage glottic can-cer. An alternative would be transoral laser surgery, but primary surgery for early glottic cancer does not include neck dissection due to the low predilection of glottic SCC for lymphatic spread.

3. **Answer E**

   Pharyngeal pouch (also known as Zenker's diverticulum) typically presents with symp-toms related to the oesophagus and throat. Common symptoms include regurgita-tion of undigested food, dysphagia (difficulty swallowing), halitosis (bad breath) and aspiration which can lead to pneumonia. Other symptoms might include a sensation of a lump in the throat, coughing, and a change in voice. Pharyngeal pouch is not associated with odynophagia (painful swallowing), which may suggest an alternate or additional diagnosis, e.g. malignancy.

4. **Answer D**

   Vocal cord nodules are benign lesions of the lamina propria often caused by vocal overuse or abuse. By altering the vibratory properties and mucosal wave of the vocal folds they may result in hoarseness or pitch and loudness perturbations. Treatment includes voice therapy and practising good vocal hygiene.

5. **Answer B**

   Intensity modulated radiation therapy (IMRT) is a highly advanced form of radiotherapy used in the treatment of head and neck squamous cell carcinoma (SCC) and other malignancies. IMRT employs computer-controlled linear accelerators to deliver precise radiation doses to a malignant tumour or specific areas within the tumour. This tech-nique allows for the radiation dose to conform more precisely to the three-dimensional (3D) shape of the tumour, thereby minimising the dose to surrounding normal critical structures. By doing so, IMRT can reduce treatment toxicity and potentially result in fewer side effects compared with conventional radiotherapy techniques. This high level of control makes IMRT a crucial tool in the modern treatment of head and neck SCC, for which the proximity of vital structures necessitates precise targeting to both ensure effective treatment and minimise harm. Particle therapy is a form of external beam radiotherapy that uses neutrons, protons or heavy ions, unlike IMRT which uses X-rays to deliver radiation to the tumour.

6. **Answer B**

Oral lichen planus (OLP) is a T-cell mediated chronic inflammatory condition that can persist for many years. The malignant transformation rate of oral lichen planus has been reported in various studies with a range typically between 0.4% and 5%. The risk may be higher in erosive or atrophic forms, and in individuals with additional risk factors such as tobacco or alcohol use. Management consists of the elimination of potential risk factors, and topical medication such as benzydamine or corticosteroid mouthwash or gels to reduce symptoms. Systemic steroids may be used in cases that do not respond to topical therapy. Second-line therapies can be considered in OLP recalcitrant to steroids, including calcineurin inhibitors (e.g. cyclosporine), or other immunosuppressants such as azathioprine or mycophenolate mofetil.

7. **Answer E**

SCC is a common type of skin cancer that can occur due to prolonged exposure to ultraviolet (UV) radiation, either from sunlight or from tanning beds or lamps. Cutaneous SCC of the head and neck, including the pinna, has a predilection for regional metastasis to intraparotid lymph nodes. Nodal metastasis to the parotid gland from cutaneous SCC accounts for up to 79% of all parotid metastases with 15% of advanced SCC (>T2) having regional metastases (neck or parotid).

Risk factors for parotid metastasis from cutaneous SCC include primary tumour size >2 cm, tumour thickness >4 mm, incomplete excision margin (<4 mm), recurrent or previously treated tumour, tumour in close anatomical proximity to the parotid, e.g. ear/temporal, high grade or desmoplastic lesion, perineural or lymphovascular invasion, advanced age and Immunosuppression.

Yii RSL, Chai SC, Wan Sulaiman WA, Mat Zain MAB. Cutaneous squamous cell carcinoma with secondary parotid metastasis: a case report. AME Case Rep. 2023 Jan 16;7:4.

8. **Answer C**

Given the patient's demographic, symptoms and the findings on flexible nasal endoscopy, nasopharyngeal carcinoma (NPC) is the most likely diagnosis. NPC has a striking geographic variation in incidence, being more common in individuals from East Asia and Africa, likely resulting from genetic, dietary and viral factors.

Based on the World Health Organization criteria NPC can be classified into three subtypes: keratinising squamous cell carcinoma, or non-keratinising carcinoma (subclassified into differentiated and undifferentiated non-keratinising carcinoma) and basaloid squamous cell carcinoma. Non-keratinising carcinoma is more common in the high-incidence population.

9. **Answer A**

Spread of disease to involve the parapharyngeal space, medial or lateral pterygoid muscle results in a T classification of T2 according to the eighth edition of TNM staging by the American Joint Committee on Cancer. T3 disease involves bony structures of the skull base, cervical vertebrae, pterygoid structures and/or paranasal sinuses, and T4 disease involves intracranial extension, cranial nerve involvement or involvement of the hypopharynx, orbit, parotid gland and/or soft tissue extension beyond the lateral surface of the lateral pterygoid muscle.

10. Answer B

Melkersson-Rosenthal syndrome, also known as orofacial granulomatosis, is a rare neurological disorder of uncertain aetiology characterised by recurring facial paralysis, swelling of the face and lips and development of folds and furrows in the tongue. This syndrome can manifest as a recurrent, intermittent condition, with the facial nerve palsy and tongue changes being characteristic features. Treatment includes non-steroidal anti-inflammatories, systemic and intra-lesional corticosteroids and immuno-suppressants. Surgery may be considered in cases of orofacial swelling refractory to medical management.

11. Answer E

From superficial to deep, the vocal cord consists of the epithelium, superficial lamina propria, intermediate lamina propria, deep lamina propria and vocalis/thyroarytenoid muscle.

The European Laryngological Society classification of endoscopic cordectomies consists of eight types:

- Subepithelial cordectomy (type I, resection of the epithelium sparing the vocal ligament and vocalis)
- Subligamental cordectomy (type II, resection of the epithelium, Reinke's space and vocal ligament)
- Transmuscular cordectomy (type III, resection through vocalis muscle, sparing at least part of the cord)
- Total cordectomy (type IV)
- Extended cordectomy (type Va, includes contralateral vocal fold and the anterior commissure)
- Extended cordectomy (type Vb, includes the arytenoid)
- Extended cordectomy (type Vc, includes the subglottis)
- Extended cordectomy (type Vd, includes the ventricle)

The choice of cordectomy depends on the tumour thickness, location and possibility of getting clear margins. If the tumour involves a phonatory segment, if it is deep (involving vocalis muscle), if there is difficult transoral access, or if it involves anterior commissure where complete resection cannot be assured, the procedure should be abandoned and the patient should be offered radiotherapy which offers the same survival outcome as surgery and better functional outcomes (voice). It is important to try to avoid dual modality treatment, for example performing transoral laser surgery and removing part of the vocalis and adjuvant radiotherapy due to incomplete resection. In a professional voice user, such as an actor, radiotherapy should be considered first-line for an early-stage laryngeal cancer given the superior voice outcomes.

Remacle, M., Eckel, H., Antonelli, A. et al. Endoscopic cordectomy. a proposal for a classification by the Working Committee, European Laryngological Society. *European Archives of Oto-Rhino-Laryngology* 257, 227–231 (2000).

12. Answer D

The symptoms of hoarseness and noisy breathing following blunt trauma to the neck are indicative of a laryngo-tracheal injury. This type of injury can cause disruption of the laryngotracheal skeleton and can result in delayed oedema.

13. Answer A

The Schaefer classification is used to categorise and describe the severity of laryngeal injuries. It provides a structured approach to assess the extent of injury which is crucial for determining the appropriate management plan. The classification system is as follows:

1) Minor endolaryngeal haematomas or lacerations without detectable fractures
2) More severe oedema, haematoma, minor mucosal disruption without exposed cartilage or non-displaced fractures
3) Massive oedema, large mucosal lacerations, exposed cartilage, displaced fractures of vocal cord immobility
4) Same as group 3 but more severe with disruption of anterior larynx, unstable fractures, two or more fracture lines or severe mucosal injuries
5) Complete laryngotracheal separation

A more pragmatic approach classifies laryngeal injuries into stable and unstable airways. Unstable airways require a definitive airway, usually via emergent tracheostomy or cricothyrotomy before any additional investigations. Patients with a stable airway may be further assessed via flexible nasendoscopy and/or imaging.

14. Answer B

Paradoxical vocal cord dysfunction (also known as inducible laryngeal obstruction) is the inappropriate adduction of the vocal cords during inhalation resulting in respiratory distress and inspiratory stridor. Patients typically present multiple times to the ED with similar symptoms that do not respond to adrenaline or bronchodilators, but tend to resolve spontaneously. Flexible laryngoscopy can be used to detect paradoxical vocal fold adduction. Spirometry may show flattening of the inspiratory or inspiratory and expiratory limbs of the flow volume loops. Treatment includes speech therapy, breathing techniques, management of triggers, e.g. gastroesophageal reflux, and rarely, vocal cord Botox injections.

15. Answer E

The combination of a unilateral headache/otalgia, jaw claudication, scalp tenderness (prominence and tenderness over the superficial temporal artery may be found), intermittent diplopia and a raised ESR is highly suggestive of temporal arteritis (giant cell arteritis, GCA). This condition is a vasculitis (nodular granulomatous inflammation) affecting large to medium-sized arteries in the elderly. GCA requires prompt diagnosis and treatment to prevent complications, including vision loss, most commonly secondary to Arteritic Anterior Ischemic Optic Neuropathy (AAION).

16. Answer C

Trigeminal neuralgia is characterised by sharp severe paroxysms of pain affecting the face and head in the distribution of the trigeminal nerve. It is caused by demyelination, usually at a site of vascular compression of the nerve.

17. Answer B

Given that the abnormality is found at the level of the supraglottis, sarcoidosis is the most likely cause of this abnormality according to the mnemonic S—A—W indicating the anatomical locations commonly affected by certain autoimmune or inflammatory conditions.

Supraglottis   – Sarcoidosis
Glottis   – Amyloidosis
Subglottis   – Wegener's (Granulomatosis with polyangiitis)

18. Answer E

Epstein-Barr virus (EBV) is known to be associated with various conditions including T-cell lymphoma, Burkitt's lymphoma, infectious mononucleosis and nasopharyngeal carcinoma. Hairy cell leukaemia is a variant of chronic lymphocytic leukaemia and is not associated with EBV.

19. Answer E

Modern preoperative investigations including CT, Sestamibi and ultrasound have reduced the need for four gland neck exploration. However, an understanding of the embryology of the parathyroid glands is important when a gland cannot be initially located. The parathyroid glands derive from the endoderm of the third and fourth pharyngeal pouches. The third pharyngeal pouch gives rise to the inferior parathyroid glands, while the superior parathyroids arise from the fourth pharyngeal pouch. Aberrant locations of the inferior parathyroid glands include the thymus gland or superior mediastinum or less commonly inside the carotid sheath or thyroid gland. The position of the inferior glands is more likely to be variable than that of the superior glands. Ectopic superior glands are most commonly found retropharyngeal/retroesophageal.

20. Answer D

The superior parathyroid glands arise from the fourth pharyngeal pouch during embryological development and are typically located superior to the inferior thyroid artery and posterolaterally to the recurrent laryngeal nerve. In contrast, the inferior parathyroids are superficial to the recurrent laryngeal nerve.

21. Answer C

The most likely cause of the neck swelling in this patient is multinodular thyroid goitre. This condition is more prevalent in certain geographic areas where there is a deficiency of iodine. It is typical for the swelling to progress over many years without other symptoms of thyroid disease.

22. Answer A

The pharyngeal arches 1 through 4 are responsible for the anatomical development of the tongue, specifically the mucosal surface of the tongue. Arch 1 forms the anterior two thirds of the tongue, arches 2, 3 and 4 form the posterior third, and arch 4 forms the epiglottis and adjacent regions. The intrinsic and extrinsic tongue musculature are derived from the occipital somites.

23. Answer C

The history is suggestive of hereditary angioedema which is caused by a deficiency or dysfunction of C1 esterase inhibitor leading to an overproduction of bradykinin. This results in increased vascular permeability and oedema. Mast cell tryptase can be useful if allergy or anaphylaxis is suspected.

24. Answer C

The bony landmark at the intersection of the coronal and sagittal suture lines, where the frontal bone and two parietal bones meet, is known as the bregma.

25. Answer B

The pterion is formed at the junction where the frontal, parietal, temporal and sphenoid bones meet. This area is clinically significant due to its proximity to the middle meningeal artery and injury to this region can lead to an Extradural haematoma.

26. Answer D

The lesser petrosal nerve is not a branch of the facial nerve. It is associated with the glossopharyngeal nerve (CN IX). The other options listed are branches of the facial nerve (CN VII).

27. Answer D

Oesophageal achalasia is characterised by a loss of ganglion cells in myenteric plexus (Auerbach's plexus), which leads to a failure of relaxation of the lower oesophageal sphincter and a loss of peristalsis in the oesophagus, making it difficult to swallow food. Oesophageal manometry reveals failure of the lower oesophageal sphincter with high pressure. Chagas disease or American trypanosomiasis is a chronic parasitic disease caused by *Trypanosoma cruzi*. Chronic Chagas disease is associated with achalasia via parasitic damage to the oesophageal myenteric plexus. *Trypanosoma brucei* infection is associated with African trypanosomiasis (sleeping sickness).

28. Answer E

The symptoms described, including abnormal winging of the scapula, are indicative of damage to the long thoracic nerve which innervates the serratus anterior muscle. The long thoracic nerve arises from the anterior rami of cervical nerves C5, C6 and C7.

29. Answer C

The symptoms described by the patient, including numbness and altered sensation on the anterior two thirds of the tongue along with a loss of taste sensation, are characteristic of an injury to the lingual nerve. The lingual nerve provides general somatic afferent innervation (sensation) to the anterior two thirds of the tongue and carries taste fibres from the same region via the chorda tympani. It is a branch of the mandibular division of the trigeminal nerve (V3). Injury to the lingual nerve can occur during surgical procedures in the vicinity of the submandibular gland given its anatomical proximity to the gland.

30. Answer C

Thy3f or follicular lesion of undetermined significance is a categorisation used for thyroid nodules when the cytological findings are suspicious but not definitive for malignancy. The Royal College of Pathologists Guidance indicates that the malignancy risk for Thy3f nodules is estimated to be 15–30%.

31. Answer B

The external branch of the superior laryngeal nerve innervates the cricothyroid muscle, which plays a crucial role in pitch modulation by tensing the vocal folds. Injury to this nerve can result in the inability to reach higher notes while singing, though conversational voice may remain unaffected.

32. Answer D

It is imperative that the mobility of the vocal cords is accurately assessed following and prior to further thyroid surgery because a postoperative bilateral vocal cord palsy is an airway emergency generally requiring a tracheostomy. In the scenario presented in the question, the surgeon should delay completion surgery until the vocal cord palsy recovers. However, if it does not recover, a decision should be made with the patient regarding the risks of completion thyroidectomy versus interval ultrasound surveillance. Completion thyroidectomy should generally be undertaken within 2–3 months; hence it would be most appropriate to rediscuss the case at the thyroid MDT. Performing surgery with untrialled equipment in difficult cases is not recommended.

33. Answer A

This presentation is consistent with Ortner's syndrome that results from a recurrent laryngeal palsy, typically on the left, in the context of cardiovascular disease. The most common cardiac abnormality is mitral stenosis that results in left atrial enlargement. The anatomy and innervation of the laryngeal muscles are fundamental knowledge for managing patients with voice disorders. The recurrent laryngeal nerve innervates all intrinsic muscles of the larynx except the cricothyroid muscle, which is innervated by the external branch of the superior laryngeal nerve.

34. Answer B

The history is consistent with salivary gland/duct caliculi. Ultrasound scanning is the preferred initial investigation for suspected salivary gland calculi because it is non-invasive and readily available and can detect stones as small as 2 mm. Additionally, it allows for real-time imaging which can be beneficial for certain therapeutic interventions.

35. Answer D

The glossopharyngeal nerve (CN IX) is responsible for secretomotor function to the parotid gland. Its tympanic branch (Jacobson's nerve) synapses in the otic ganglion, and postganglionic fibres then travel via the auriculotemporal nerve to provide secretomotor innervation to the parotid gland. Unilateral parotid surgery does not consistently increase the risk of xerostomia.

36. Answer B

Bilateral parotid swelling may be due to systemic disease, e.g. infection, immune/autoimmune disease, or related to primary salivary gland disease, e.g. salivary stones, sialadenitis or neoplasia. Although a family history of rheumatoid arthritis may be suggestive of an autoimmune cause, the most likely cause from the information given in the question is diabetes. About 25% of patients with overt or latent diabetes (HBA1c >6%) have bilateral asymptomatic enlargement of the parotid glands.

37. Answer D

Obstructive sleep apnoea is characterised by repeated partial or complete obstruction of the upper airways during sleep. Untreated OSA in adults is associated with neurocognitive and cardiovascular morbidity. The first line-management of symptomatic adult OSA, as described in the scenario, is weight loss (if high BMI) and CPAP. In patients intolerant of CPAP, surgical options may be considered to improve CPAP compliance. For instance, in the patient in the scenario, tonsillectomy/septoplasty may be warranted.

38. Answer A

Deficiency of the mandibular or maxillary projection are a known risk factor for OSA through a reduction in the upper airway size. An inferior hyoid position, or face long in the vertical/sagittal plane, increases the length of the airway, increasing instability and the risk of airway collapse. Increased nasal resistance, increased tongue size, large tonsils and a long soft palate are additional risk factors.

39. Answer C

NICE (National Institute for Health and Care Excellence) guidelines recommend PET-CT in the setting of head and neck SCC of unknown primary, T4 nasopharyngeal carcinoma and T4 hypopharyngeal carcinoma. T4 supraglottic SCC carries a significant risk of lymph node metastasis but is not by itself an indication for pre-treatment staging PET-CT.

40. Answer B

MRI with gadolinium enhancement provides superior soft tissue contrast and can better delineate the extent of the lesion, including any deep lobe extension, compared to other imaging modalities listed.

41. Answer E

Pleomorphic adenomas are especially common in the parotid gland, accounting for the majority of benign salivary gland tumours. The aetiology of pleomorphic adenoma is unknown, but the incidence of this tumour has been increasing in the last 15–20 years. Oncogenic simian virus (SV40) may play a role in the onset or progression of pleomorphic adenoma. Prior head and neck irradiation is also a risk factor for the development of these tumours.

42. Answer A

The risk of malignant transformation into carcinoma ex-pleomorphic adenoma is proportionate to the time the lesion remains in situ. The risk stands at approximately 1.5% in the first five years. The transformation into carcinoma ex-pleomorphic adenoma is a rare but serious event that justifies the recommendation for surgical excision of pleomorphic adenomas at diagnosis to mitigate this risk. Some additional risk factors for malignancy include advanced age, large size of the tumour, prior radiation therapy and recurrent tumours.

43. Answer A

CT neck and chest with contrast should be undertaken in cases of thyroid cancer with suspected retrosternal extension, tracheal compression or invasion. It should also be undertaken for patients with N1 disease and locally advanced T3–4 tumours, as is the case in this scenario. A CT without contrast is less useful to detect lower neck or upper chest nodal disease. Iodine in iodinated contrast agents may interfere with radioactive iodine (RAI) treatment, but this is usually not an issue since there is generally an interval of over 2 months between staging and RAI treatment.

A radioactive iodine uptake (RIU) test is primarily used in the evaluation of hyperthyroidism but may be used to determine whether functioning metastases are amenable to radioactive iodine therapy. Therefore, the RIU test would not be appropriate as an initial staging scan. PET-CT may be used detect local and distant recurrence after surgery/radioiodine.

44. Answer C

Mucoepidermoid carcinoma (MEC) is the most common type of salivary gland cancer and occurs with a peak incidence between 30 and 60 years of age, more commonly in females. These malignancies may exhibit slow or fast growth, forming mucous-filled cysts from the mucoepidermoid cells lining the gland. Histologically, three cell types can be defined: mucous, intermediate and squamous. Higher-grade lesions contain a larger squamous component. While they predominantly occur in the parotid gland, mucoepidermoid carcinomas can also develop in the submandibular and minor salivary glands. MEC is associated with a translocation resulting in fusion *CTRC1-MAML2* oncogene, particularly in low- and intermediate-grade tumours. Complete surgical resection with clear margins is recommended, with a neck dissection +/- radiotherapy depending on nodal status or in the case of high-grade lesions.

45. Answer C

HPV strain 16 is the most common strain associated with oropharyngeal squamous cell carcinoma. This strain, along with strain 18, significantly contributes to the development of head and neck cancers, with strain 16 being more prevalent.

46. Answer C

The tonsils are the most common sub-site for oropharyngeal squamous cell carcinoma, particularly in HPV-associated cases. The second most common sub-site is the base of the tongue. Identification of the primary tumour site is pivotal for staging, treatment planning and prognostication. The piriform fossa is a sub-site of the hypopharynx.

47. Answer D

Keratoacanthoma (KA) is a low-grade skin tumour characterised by rapid growth, followed by a period of stability, and eventually, spontaneous regression. Originating from the pilosebaceous unit, KAs predominantly arise in sun-exposed or hair-bearing areas but can also manifest in other regions, including the oral mucosa. Although histologically similar to squamous cell carcinoma, KAs are recognised as benign.

48. Answer B

The pharyngeal phase of swallowing is chiefly orchestrated by the glossopharyngeal and vagus nerves. The glossopharyngeal nerve (IX) and pharyngeal branches of the vagus nerve (X) innervate the pharynx and larynx, coordinating their actions through a swallowing centre in the brainstem. This reflexive sequence propels ingesta from the pharynx into the oesophagus, marking the transition from the oral to the pharyngeal phase of deglutition.

49. Answer C

Considering that this lesion is localised to one vocal cord with no nodal involvement or distant metastasis, the likely staging is T1aN0M0. The T1a stage denotes a carcinoma limited to one vocal cord, while N0 and M0 indicate no regional lymph node metastasis and no distant metastasis, respectively. Involvement of the false vocal fold as well as the true vocal fold indicates T2 disease. Depth of invasion is important in staging of oral cavity SCC but not other sub-sites of head and neck SCC.

50. Answer A

The auscultatory sign described, in which a gurgling sound is heard upon auscultating the soft, compressible mass in the neck, is known as Boyce's sign. This is a characteristic finding in cases of pharyngeal pouch (Zenker's diverticulum).

51. Answer C

The most likely diagnosis in this case is a laryngocele, a dilatation of the saccule of the laryngeal ventricle. This condition is commonly associated with activities that involve raised intralaryngeal pressure, such as playing brass or woodwind instruments. The symptoms can vary from mild throat irritation to more severe complications like airway obstruction. Laryngoceles can be classified as internal (with the laryngocele confined to the paraglottic space), external (saccule herniates through the thyrohyoid membrane) or mixed.

52. Answer C

The most common anatomical location for a squamous cell carcinoma (SCC) within the hypopharynx to arise is the piriform fossa. The hypopharynx extends from the level of the hyoid bone to the lower end of the cricoid cartilage and includes the post-cricoid region, piriform fossa and the posterior pharyngeal wall. About 70% of hypopharyngeal tumours originate in the piriform fossa.

53. Answer D

The ascending pharyngeal artery is the primary blood supply for a glomus jugulare tumour, which is what is suspected in this case based on the patient's symptoms and clinical findings.

54. Answer A

Surgery is the treatment of choice for malignant salivary tumours. A total parotidectomy, with preservation of the facial nerve if it is assessed as uninvolved intraoperatively, is generally recommended. Small or low-grade malignancies may be managed with a superficial parotidectomy; however this would not be appropriate in the case of an adenoid cystic carcinoma (high grade). If the facial nerve is found to be involved, then it should be resected, and the resection should be accompanied by a reconstructive procedure such as a cable graft or static sling. Resection of an uninvolved facial nerve in adenoid cystic carcinoma has not been associated with improved local control. Adjuvant radiotherapy is recommended for adenoid cystic carcinoma and for control of the neck disease (since this is advanced-stage disease, N1 and stage III).

55. Answer B

In a patient with HPV-positive or -negative SCC of unknown primary with a single involved node of 3cm or less and no radiological extra-nodal extension, single modality surgery may be considered appropriate. This would generally consist of bilateral tonsillectomy, tongue base mucosectomy and an ipsilateral selective neck dissection level 2–4.

56. Answer A

For this scenario the MRI neck, ultrasound and FNA are requested at the same time as primary investigations. This scenario describes a head and neck squamous cell carcinoma of unknown primary. Current NICE guidelines recommend the use of PET-CT (using Fludeoxyglucose, FDG-18F, which is a marker for tissue uptake of glucose) for patients with confirmed metastatic SCC in whom the primary site has not been found on examination or MRI. DOTATATE PET scans are used for the diagnosis of neuroendocrine tumours, e.g. carcinoid, paraganglioma and myeloma. An open excisional biopsy should not be used as a first-line investigation to diagnose cervical metastasis. Although the majority of head and neck cancers are sporadic there are reports of familial clustering. However, there is currently limited evidence on the role of genetic factors in the development of head and neck cancers and hence a referral to genetics is not warranted in this scenario.

57. Answer C

The most likely diagnosis in this scenario is a vocal cord cyst. Treatment often combines surgical excision and voice therapy in an MDT clinic.

58. Answer D

According to SIGN/NICE guidelines, a minimum of five episodes of symptomatic tonsillitis per year over a consecutive 2-year period is generally required to consider a patient for tonsillectomy. In this patient's case, he has had three episodes per year for two years, which does not meet the criteria.

59. Answer B

The most likely diagnosis is follicular carcinoma of the thyroid. This type of thyroid cancer is characterised by its propensity for vascular invasion. Follicular carcinoma is the second most common type of thyroid cancer. It has a unique pattern of haematogenous spread, most commonly metastasising to the lungs and bones. Treatment is dependent on size and histopathological features, and maximally will involve total thyroidectomy +/- neck dissection followed by radioactive iodine therapy.

60. Answer A

This patient has advanced nasopharyngeal cancer (T4N2Mx, stage IV). Intensity modulated radiotherapy is standard-of-care treatment with the addition of platinum chemotherapy for stage II (except T2N0), stage III and stage IV disease. Induction chemotherapy should be considered in all patients with locoregionally advanced NPC. Surgical options, either open or endoscopic, may be considered for recurrent disease if it is considered likely that clear margins can be achieved. However, this must be weighed against the risk of significant morbidity, and recurrence may also be considered for reirradiation.

61. Answer A

Gardasil is an HPV vaccine for use in the prevention of certain strains of human papillomavirus (HPV). High-risk human papilloma virus (hr-HPV) genital infection is the most common sexually transmitted infection among women. The HPV strains that Gardasil protects against are sexually transmitted, specifically HPV types 6, 11, 16 and 18. HPV types 16 and 18 cause an estimated 70% of cervical cancers, and are responsible for most HPV-induced anal, vulvar, vaginal and penile cancer cases. Cervarix protects against HPV 16 and 18. HPV types 6 and 11 cause an estimated 90% of genital warts cases and RRP.

62. Answer D

Hyperkalaemia is the most likely concern in this clinical scenario. The patient has acute tubular necrosis, a form of acute kidney injury, which hampers the kidney's ability to excrete potassium. During the maintenance phase of acute tubular necrosis, urine output is minimal, leading to the retention of potassium and hence hyperkalaemia. This is a serious complication that can lead to cardiac arrhythmias and requires immediate attention.

63. Answer B

The history of bleeding two weeks after a prior tracheostomy is highly suggestive of a tracheoinnominate fistula (TIF) whereby there is a fistulous connection between the innominate artery and the trachea. The innominate artery normally crosses the trachea between the sixth and ninth cartilage ring. Risk factors for a TIF include prolonged intubation, tracheitis, tracheostomy placed lower than the third ring and cuff over inflation. The Utley manoeuvre involves placing a finger through the incision to compress the innominate artery against the posterior sternum. This can also be achieved by overinflating the cuff. Removing the tracheostomy and replacing with a cuffed endotracheal tube that can be inflated below the bleeding site is another potential temporising solution. These measures may temporise the situation; however, definitive emergent surgical management should be undertaken, either open via sternotomy or endovascular stent placement in those who are not candidates for surgery. Local haemostatic strategies including electrocautery and packing are unlikely to be successful. Imaging studies have limited sensitivity in the diagnosis of TIF, and imaging in an unstable, bleeding patient is potentially catastrophic. Removing the tracheostomy tube and attempting to orally intubate risks losing the ability to ventilate the patient given that oral intubation is likely to be difficult in this situation (bleeding, obese).

64. Answer C

Patients undergoing Sistrunk's procedure for thyroglossal duct cyst require ultrasound to ensure the presence of normal thyroid tissue. Rarely, a thyroglossal duct cyst contains the patient's only functioning thyroid tissue.

65. Answer C

Joll's triangle is an anatomical landmark useful for identifying the external branch of the superior laryngeal nerve (EBSLN) during thyroidectomy. This triangle is bordered superiorly by the superior attachment of the strap muscles, medially by the midline and laterally by the upper pole of the thyroid gland and superior thyroid vessels. The EBSLN lies in the floor of this triangle, formed by the cricothyroid muscle. Knowledge of this anatomical landmark is crucial for avoiding injury to the EBSLN, which innervates the cricothyroid muscle and contributes to voice quality.

66. Answer A

The digastric muscle consists of two bellies united by an intermediate rounded tendon. The two bellies of the digastric muscle have different embryological origins, and are supplied by different cranial nerves. The anterior belly is derived from the first pharyngeal arch and supplied by the mylohyoid nerve, a branch of the inferior alveolar nerve, itself a branch of the mandibular division of the trigeminal nerve. The posterior belly is derived from the second pharyngeal arch and supplied by the digastric branch of the facial nerve.

67. Answer C

Psammoma bodies, orphan Annie nuclei (chromatin clearing with peripheral margination of chromatin), enlarged/irregular nuclei and intra-nuclear cytoplasmic pseudo-inclusions are characteristic of papillary thyroid carcinoma. Follicular thyroid carcinoma is typified by cuboidal epithelial cells that have capsular and vascular invasive properties. Anaplastic thyroid carcinoma has invasive sarcomatoid, giant cell or epithelial features. Oncocytic thyroid carcinoma is rich in mitochondria.

68. Answer D

Although highly effective for the management of OSA, CPAP has poor long-term compliance, typically defined as using CPAP 4 hours/night for 5 nights a week. Compliance failures primarily stem from patient comfort factors, including nasal/oral dryness, nasal irritation, claustrophobia and high device noise levels. The Muller manoeuvre requires the patient to attempt to inhale against a closed mouth and pinched nose. Using a flexible nasendoscope introduced into the hypopharynx it is possible to assess airway collapse. A positive test result means the site of upper airway obstruction is likely below the level of the soft palate and the patient will not likely benefit from oropharyngeal surgery (tonsillectomy/UVPP) in isolation. Although the high BMI, large tonsils and septal deviation in this patient may be contributing to reduced CPAP tolerability, non-surgical management should be instigated primarily.

69. Answer D

The gold standard for diagnosing a pharyngeal pouch is a barium swallow. This type of pouch, also known as Zenker's diverticulum, commonly presents in older patients with symptoms like dysphagia, regurgitation, chest infections and weight loss. Barium swallow is especially effective because it visualises the pouch and helps in planning subsequent treatment, such as endoscopic stapling or open surgery. Early identification and treatment are crucial to prevent complications such as aspiration pneumonia.

70. Answer D

Reconstruction of large hypopharyngeal defects following laryngopharyngectomy has classically been performed using jejunal or radial forearm free flap. The best swallowing outcomes are reported for the jejunal free flap because although it is not innervated, it retains peristaltic action. More recently, the anterolateral thigh flap (ALT) has been increasingly used given its superior voice outcomes and greater familiarity to current reconstructive surgeons. The deltopectoral flap is a regional cutaneous flap and not a free flap. It is a versatile flap for head and neck reconstruction and may still be used in cases unsuitable for microvascular anastomoses.

71. Answer B

Botulinum toxin A is most effectively administered intradermally for treating Frey's syndrome. This method has been shown to improve symptoms significantly and enhance the patient's quality of life. Although symptoms might recur, repeat injections remain effective.

72. Answer B

Frey's syndrome occurs due to aberrant reinnervation of postganglionic parasympathetic neurons to nearby denervated sweat glands and cutaneous blood vessels. In essence, parasympathetic fibres that originally innervated the parotid gland now stimulate the sweat glands in the skin, resulting in symptoms like sweating and flushing upon mastication. The neurotransmitter responsible for mediating this action is acetylcholine.

73. Answer C

The patient has metastatic papillary thyroid cancer, and the most comprehensive approach would be to perform a total thyroidectomy with a lateral neck dissection. Due the metastatic nature of the cancer at presentation, radioactive iodine therapy should also be considered as part of the treatment plan.

74. Answer C

The anterior branch of the middle meningeal artery is most likely the culprit in an extradural haematoma. This artery traverses the foramen spinosum, which is found in the greater wing of the sphenoid bone.

75. Answer D

Given his long history of smoking and symptoms like voice fatigue and breathlessness, there would be a high suspicion of a vocal cord palsy due to a lung malignancy. A left-sided pleural effusion on the chest X-ray further supports this. Immediate CT scanning and consultations with specialists in speech and language therapy, as well as chest medicine, are warranted. Smoking cessation is critical in this case.

76. Answer C

CT from the skull base to the diaphragm is the most appropriate first-line investigation in order to exclude lesions along the course of the vagus and recurrent laryngeal nerves. MRI brain is sometimes useful to exclude central causes but is not a first-line investigation. These patients do require input from speech and language therapists to ensure they are not aspirating and for compensatory exercises.

77. Answer B

The appearance of the tongue is most likely a form of chronic atrophic oral candidiasis, known as median rhomboid glossitis. Treatment can involve antifungal medication, usually in the form of capsules or tablets, and good oral hygiene.

78. Answer A

The treatment of T4 N1–3 M0 supraglottic cancer is a total laryngectomy with bilateral neck dissection +/- reconstruction and post-operative radiotherapy +/- chemotherapy. Primary chemoradiotherapy may be considered in patients with low volume disease with minimal cartilage invasion and preserved laryngeal function; hence it would not be appropriate in this scenario. T4b tumours invade the prevertebral space, encase the carotid or mediastinal structures and are generally unresectable and patients should be offered primary radiotherapy +/- chemotherapy or best supportive care.

79. Answer B

The presence of antibodies to desmoglein-3 is indicative of pemphigus, an autoimmune blistering disease affecting the skin and mucous membranes. Treatment often involves oral steroids and possibly other immunomodulators.

80. Answer A

The Friedman staging system (stage I/II/III) is determined by the Friedman tongue position (grade 1–4), tonsil size (grade 1–4) and BMI (greater or less than 40). Patients with a Friedman stage I have an over 80% chance of surgical success with UVPP. A patient with a tongue position revealing the uvula and tonsils/pillars (Friedman tongue position grade 1), small tonsils and a low BMI would be the most favourable surgical candidate. Friedman stage II and III patients have a poor rate of UVPP surgical success.

81. Answer A

The most cited criteria for success of sleep surgery are those proposed by Sher et al. These authors defined surgical success for OSA surgery as a reduction in baseline apnoea-hypopnea index (AHI) of more than 50% and a post-operative AHI of fewer than 20 events/hour. Subsequently, other authors have proposed modified versions, such as the SLEEP GOAL criteria, that use a composite measure of snoring improvement, latency of sleep onset, Epworth sleepiness score, CPAP usage, systolic blood pressure, BMI, AHI, oxygenation and quality of life score. However, in the OSA literature and clinical practice the Sher criteria are the most commonly used. According to these criteria, surgery in this patient has been successful and further surgery is not warranted.

Sher AE, Schechtman KB, Piccirillo JF (1996) The efficacy of surgical modifications of the upper airway in adults with obstructive sleep apnea syndrome. *Sleep* 19(2):156–177

Pang, K.P., Rotenberg, B.W. The SLEEP GOAL as a success criteria in obstructive sleep apnea therapy. *Eur Arch Otorhinolaryngol* 273, 1063–1065 (2016)

82. Answer A

Plain film radiography is readily available and can diagnose radio-opaque upper aerodigestive tract foreign bodies prior to definitive management with rigid or flexible pharyngo-oesophagoscopy.

83. Answer D

The tumour in the left tonsil is 2.5 cm, fitting the T2 classification. The neck node is 6.5 cm, which is classified as N3. There are no distant metastases, making it M0. Therefore, the MDT staging for this tumour would be T2N3M0.

84. Answer B

The stylopharyngeus muscle is innervated by the glossopharyngeal nerve (cranial nerve IX). This muscle acts to elevate the larynx and pharynx and dilate the pharynx, facilitating swallowing.

85. Answer D

Renal function tests are crucial in this case to assess for dehydration, which is a common cause of salivary gland swelling and dysfunction. Ensuring proper hydration can alleviate the symptoms.

86. Answer B

A CO_2 laser is most appropriate for resection of oral and tongue lesions. It offers precise cutting and has been widely used in the management of oral premalignant disorders.

87. Answer C

Jitter represents the cycle-to-cycle variability in the period duration of the acoustic voice signal. It serves as a measure of the micro-instability of vocal cord vibrations and can be used to detect voice pathologies.

88. Answer B

Oral candidiasis is a mycosis (yeast/fungal infection) of Candida species on the mucous membranes of the mouth. HIV-related immunosuppression predisposes to oral candidiasis infection.

Candida albicans is the most commonly implicated organism in this condition. *C. albicans* is carried in the mouths of about 50% of the world's population as a normal component of the oral microbiota. This candidal carriage state is not considered pathological, but when Candida species invade host tissues, oral candidiasis can occur. This change usually constitutes an opportunistic infection because of local (i.e., mucosal) or systemic factors altering host immunity.

89. Answer D

The history of smoking, raspy voice, and the presence of white lesions on both sides of the vocal cords is consistent with leukoplakia. This condition is often a presentation of dysplasia and 25% of leukoplakic lesions are dysplastic. Malignant transformation rate is 14% over 5.8 years and severity of dysplasia correlates with likelihood of malignant transformation. Approximately 30% of severe dysplasia undergoes malignant transformation, in contrast to 10% of mild to moderate dysplastic lesions.

Surgical excision should be performed and reduces this risk but follow-up is required. In terms of management, severe dysplasia and carcinoma in situ should be regarded as synonymous. Low-risk lesions, which includes patients who have mild or moderate dysplasia with no visible lesion, with hoarseness, and who do not smoke, can be followed up for 6 months. High-risk lesions should be followed up for 5 years in a head and neck clinic, in the same way as a T1 glottic SCC.

90. Answer B

MEN2A is an inherited disease caused by a mutation in the *RET* gene. It is characterised by medullary carcinoma of the thyroid, pheochromocytoma and parathyroid hyperplasia or adenomas. Thyroidectomy is recommended by 5 years old, and genetic screening for the family is suggested once a diagnosis has been made. The possibility of pheochromocytomas in this disease means that patients must be screened for this pre-operatively because this would need to be managed first, to make a general anaesthetic safe.

91. Answer C

A careful infectious disease history should be taken and this should be jointly managed with the microbiology team, with diphtheria being a potential cause of the grey adherent plaque and sepsis. Diphtheria anti-toxin should be administered along with antimicrobials.

92. Answer E

A non-contrast CT neck done without delay will aid decision making and potentially avoid an unnecessary general anaesthetic for an elderly co-morbid patient. Sharp foreign bodies should be removed as quickly as possible under direct vision under general anaesthetic.

93. Answer D

In the absence of airway compromise currently it would be reasonable to trial steroids to see if this will aid the shortness of breath for this palliative patient. If a tracheostomy can be avoided this would likely be in her best interests.

94. Answer B

An ALT, RFFF or jejunal free flap would be reasonable reconstructive options for this patient; a RFFF is precluded by the Allen test showing the patient is dependent on their radial artery for arterial blood flow, previous bowel cancer and previous abdominal surgery make a jejunal free flap more challenging and a RIG will mean a gastric pull-up is not an option.

95. Answer D

Depth of invasion (DOI), defined as the vertical distance between the basement membrane and the deepest part of the tumour, is a strong predictor of lymph node metastasis. It therefore forms part of the T classification in the eighth edition of the AJCC TNM staging system for oral cavity cancers, with T1 cancers having a DOI of <5 mm, T2 cancers having a DOI of 5–10 mm (or any tumour 2–4 cm diameter with a DOI <10 mm) and T3 cancers having a DOI of >10 mm (or any tumour >4 cm diameter). Depth of invasion is not an indication for adjuvant chemotherapy.

96. **Answer D**

    Familial adenomatous polyposis (FAP) causes widespread polyposis throughout the colon and rectum, and results in an increased risk of colorectal cancer. Two percent of patients with FAP develop papillary thyroid carcinoma, the vast majority of these being female.

97. **Answer A**

    MEN2B is caused by a germline mutation in the *RET* proto-oncogene and results in medullary thyroid carcinoma, phaeochromocytoma, a Marfanoid body habitus, mucosal neuromas and gastrointestinal ganglioneuromas. The most common eye sign of MEN2B is thickening of the corneal nerves, in addition to eyelid and conjunctival neuromas. Over 50% of cases of MEN2B are caused by sporadic germline mutations, i.e. not hereditary.

98. **Answer E**

    Parastomal recurrence is associated with all of the options except free flap reconstruction of the pharynx. It can be classified using the Sisson classification, with early recurrences limited to the tracheal stoma and upper oesophagus being amenable to surgical resection, but in general the prognosis is poor.

99. **Answer B**

    Oral lichen planus is a chronic condition thought to be autoimmune. If painless it does not need to be treated, but painful lesions can be treated with topical steroids. Any suspicious lesions should be biopsied to rule out dysplasia or malignancy, but surgical excision is not appropriate. In some cases, drugs such as azathioprine and methotrexate are used but these are not first-line treatments.

100. **Answer E**

    Chyle leak can be confirmed by testing drain fluid for triglycerides and chylomicrons. It is vital that drain output is accurately recorded, and fluid and electrolyte status is monitored closely and corrected. Simple measures include nursing head up, prescribing laxatives to avoid straining, and instigating a medium chain fatty acid diet. High volume or persistent leaks may require surgical exploration, treatment with octreotide or ligation/embolisation of the thoracic duct.

101. **Answer D**

    In penetrating neck trauma with no hard signs of airway or vascular injury, a CT angiogram should be performed following initial assessment. In this case, the patient is stable with no hard signs of vascular injury necessitating immediate transfer to theatre and surgical exploration, and the information from the CT will be useful in planning surgical exploration of the neck.

102. **Answer C**

    An aberrant right subclavian artery passes posterior to the oesophagus and is associated with a non-recurrent right recurrent laryngeal nerve which passes horizontally from the vagus nerve in the neck towards the larynx. This is at risk of injury during thyroid surgery.

CHAPTER 3: PAEDIATRICS

1. **You admit a 1-year-old boy with acute otitis media and fevers. What is the first clinical sign of intracranial infection?**
   A Neck stiffness
   B Vomiting
   C Irritability
   D Seizure
   E Papilloedema

2. **You are working in the paediatric ENT clinic and are seeing a 6-year-old boy with bilateral sensorineural hearing loss. You notice from the case records he has a recent abnormal perchlorate discharge test organised by your consultant colleague. Which syndrome does he likely have?**
   A CHARGE syndrome
   B Pendred syndrome
   C Goldenhar syndrome
   D VACTERL
   E Multiple endocrine neoplasia type 2

3. **You are called to the NICU to evaluate a 2-day-old term baby who was noted to have respiratory distress. What is the most common cause of nasal obstruction in a neonate?**
   A Pyriform aperture stenosis
   B Neonatal rhinitis
   C Nasal dermoid
   D Adenoid hypertrophy
   E Dacryocystocele

4. **You see a 5-year-old boy in clinic with a right preauricular mass. His mother tells you it has become infected twice and he has received antibiotics from his GP. You organise an ultrasound that suggests a first branchial cleft cyst. You decide to surgically resect the cyst using a facial nerve monitor. What is the associated nerve of the first branchial arch?**
   A Vagus nerve
   B Hypoglossal nerve
   C Accessory nerve
   D Facial nerve
   E Trigeminal nerve

5. **You review a 10-year-old girl in the outpatient clinic. On examination you note a solitary median maxillary incisor. You should consider which associated brain abnormality?**
   A Congenital hydrocephalus
   B Dandy Walker malformation
   C Arnold Chiari malformation
   D Holoprosencephaly
   E Interhemispheric cyst

6. **A mother brings her 10-month-old child to clinic. She is concerned that after feeding the baby cries and is irritated. She has also noticed that feeding can bring on neck and back spasms. What is the most likely diagnosis?**
   A Wilson's disease
   B Sandifer syndrome
   C West syndrome
   E Infantile colic
   E Subglottic stenosis

7. **Which of these conditions is associated with premature fusion of the coronal cranial sutures?**
   A Brachycephaly
   B Scaphocephaly
   C Plagiocephaly
   D Kleeblattschaedel
   E Trigonocephaly

DOI: 10.1201/9781003455059-3

8. **You review a newborn on NICU. You review the chart and note the baby has feeding difficulties, a cleft palate, tetralogy of Fallot and thymic aplasia. The most likely diagnosis is:**
   A CHARGE syndrome
   B VACTERL
   C DiGeorge syndrome
   D Zellweger syndrome
   E Cri du Chat

9. **You are about to perform a cortical mastoidectomy on a 15 kg 2-year-old boy with a mastoid abscess. You inform the anaesthetist you are about to inject some lignocaine with adrenaline before incision. The anaesthetist asks how much you are planning to give. What is the maximum amount of 2% lignocaine with 1:80,000 adrenaline that you can give?**
   A 2 ml
   B 4 ml
   C 5 ml
   D 10 ml
   E 15 ml

10. **You are called to the ED to review a 3-year-old boy with a postauricular swelling and discharging ear. He is febrile and has vomited. What is the most appropriate first step in management?**
    A IV access
    B CT temporal bone scan
    C MRI brain with contrast
    D Notify theatres of an emergency case
    E CT temporal bone scan with contrast

11. **A 5-month-old boy is brought to clinic for frequent noisy breathing. The mother reports that the child has been treated for pneumonia three times in his life and had always been a "colicky" baby. Examination reveals biphasic stridor and a mild tracheal tug. Diagnostic rigid laryngo-tracheo-bronchoscopy (LTB) is performed revealing anterior-only compression of the trachea. What is the most likely diagnosis?**
    A Double aortic arch

    B Pulmonary artery stenosis
    C Tracheoesphageal fistula
    D Aberrant innominate artery
    E Tracheomalacia

12. **A 13-year-old boy comes to clinic with reports of frequent large-volume epistaxis and nasal obstruction. On a previous visit to ED for epistaxis his nose was examined resulting in considerable bleeding. He refuses examination in the clinic room today. What is the next appropriate step?**
    A Arrange contrast-enhanced CT sinuses
    B Continue with examination
    C Arrange examination under general anaesthesia
    D Arrange MRI sinuses and brain
    E Prescribe Naseptin for 7 days with 3-month follow-up

13. **You are called to the ED to see a 5-year-old girl with a large antero-lateral neck swelling. She is febrile and looks unwell. There is a mild stertor when she lies on the bed. You explain to her male carer that she needs urgent surgery to drain the neck abscess. He tells you he is the partner of the child's mother and not her legal guardian. What is next most appropriate step?**
    A Try to telephone the mother to establish consent
    B Contact Trust legal advisor
    C Proceed without consent
    D Ask the male carer to sign the consent form
    E Manage the neck abscess medically

14. **You review a 1-week-old baby with a cleft palate on NICU. They have been requiring respiratory support and a nasopharyngeal airway. Regarding the Pierre Robin sequence (PRS), which statement is correct?**
    A PRS has a known single genetic abnormality
    B PRS results from micrognathia leading to tongue displacement

C PRS is the most common cause of primary macroglossia

D PRS-associated cleft palate is typically Y-shaped

E PRS is associated with subglottic stenosis

15. A 14-year-old girl comes to ED with a 4-day history of sore throat, odynophagia and fever. Examination reveals bilateral large, non-exudative, erythematous tonsils. The neck is soft and mobile. What is the most likely causative organism?

A *Streptococcus pyogenes*

B *Haemophilus influenzae*

C *Rhinovirus*

D *Staphylococcus aureus*

E *Fusobacterium necrophorum*

16. You are called urgently to ED to see a 3-year-old boy who has been repeatedly vomiting after ingesting a household cleaning product. On examination he is clearly in pain and respiratory distress. There is evidence of surgical emphysema over the neck and upper chest. Which is the most appropriate first investigation?

A CT neck and chest without contrast

B CT neck and chest with contrast

C Oesophagogastroduodenoscopy (OGD) performed by the paediatric/gastroenterology team

D Rigid oesphagoscopy

E Flexible nasoendoscopy

17. A 6-year-old boy comes to the ED with a swollen right eye and nasal discharge. When you see him he is playing with his sister. A CT sinus is performed revealing pansinusitis and a 0.8 cm subperiosteal abscess lateral to the lamina paparycea. The eye has full range of movement and the visual acuity is normal. The most appropriate next step in management is:

A Obtain MRI sinuses and brain

B Emergency external drainage

C Commence 24 hours IV antibiotics

D Discharge on 7 days oral antibiotics

E Emergency endoscopic sinus surgery and orbital decompression

18. An 8-year-old girl is playing with her brother and sustains a nasal trauma. One week later she presents to the ED with bilateral nasal obstruction and fever. Examination reveals a septal abscess. The most appropriate next step in management is:

A Needle aspiration under local anaesthetic

B Incision and drainage under general anaesthetic

C Needle aspiration under general anaesthetic

D Incision and drainage under local anaesthetic

E Intranasal packing and admission for IV antibiotics

19. You are seeing a 2-month-old baby in clinic. Her mother has concerns over a new and growing raised, red lesion on the baby's left cheek. The baby is otherwise well and feeding and growing normally. Which statement is true regarding the most likely diagnosis?

A The baby is at increased risk of laryngomalacia

B The lesion is likely to express Glut-2 transporter

C The baby is at increased risk of subglottic haemangioma

D The baby requires an urgent airway endoscopy in theatre

E Propranolol is an appropriate treatment for this condition

20. You are called urgently to attend the ED to evaluate a 3-year-old girl who was found coughing in her playroom by her older sister. The ED have performed a chest X-ray revealing a radio-opaque foreign body at the level of the hyoid appearing to be in the upper oesophagus on the lateral view. The ED doctor tells you he thinks he can see a "double ring sign". The vital signs are stable and there is no airway distress. Oropharyngeal and chest examination

are normal. Which is the next most appropriate step in management?

A Flexible nasendoscopy
B Flexible bronchoscopy
C Rigid endoscopy
D CT chest and abdomen
E Recommend referral to paediatric surgeons

21. You are called to the ED to see a 5-month-old boy presenting as an emergency with increased work of breathing, and biphasic stridor. The oxygen saturations are currently 100% on room air. Flexible nasendoscopy is performed revealing the lesion shown in Figure 3.1. Which of these statements is true?

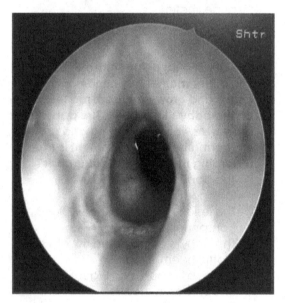

Figure 3.1 Throat.

A 50% of these lesions will self-regress by the age of 5
B A tracheostomy is indicated to protect the airway
C Propranolol should be started immediately
D Steroids and nebulised adrenaline are not indicated in this situation
E Surgery is associated with superior outcomes than medical management in primary cases

22. A 4-month-old female had a patent ductus arteriosus repair performed at 6 weeks old. Subsequently she has had a breathy, dysphonic cry. There is no respiratory distress and no aspiration concern. There is no documentation in her surgical notes as to whether the recurrent laryngeal nerve was injured. You perform a flexible nasendoscopy and laryngoscopy on her and she has a left-sided vocal cord palsy. How should you manage this patient?

A Laryngeal reinnervation procedure
B Watchful waiting
C Type 1 thyroplasty: medialisation laryngoplasty
D Injection laryngoplasty—medialisation of the vocal cord using a 'filler'
E Nasogastric tube placement

23. A 5-year-old child has a right-sided vocal cord palsy and a laryngeal reinnervation procedure is being considered. Which nerve is preferred for grafting?

A Vagus nerve
B Ansa cervicalis
C Posterior great auricular nerve
D Phrenic nerve
E Sural nerve

24. You review a 3-year-old boy in clinic. His parents have concerns about the appearance of his ear and his hearing. Examination reveals a unilateral grade 2 microtia and an atretic external auditory canal. A CT temporal bones reveals a sclerotic mastoid, an aerated middle ear space, a disrupted malleo-incudal complex and evidence of a malformed stapes. The rest of the temporal bone appears normal. Regarding surgery, which of these is correct?

A The patient is a good candidate for atresiaplasty
B The patient is a moderate candidate for atresiaplasty
C The patient is a poor candidate for atresiaplasty

D Correction of microtia should be undertaken at the same time as atresiaplasty

E Atresiaplasty is contraindicated in the presence of microtia

25. You review a 7-year-old boy in clinic with concerns regarding his tonsils. He reports some mild sore throat and occasional choking on food. Examination reveals large tonsils with the right side being larger than the left. Examination of the neck reveals a few small lymph nodes. The next best step in management is:
   A Observe for 6 weeks and reassess
   B MRI neck
   C CT neck
   D List for diagnostic tonsillectomy
   E Refer to haematology

26. The daily maintenance fluid requirement for a 20 kg child is:
   A 1500 ml
   B 1000 ml
   C 2000 ml
   D 2500 ml
   E 3000 ml

27. You review an 8-year-old boy in clinic who has a background of cerebral palsy and severe neurodevelopmental delay. His mother explains that his drooling has become more problematic and now requires multiple clothing changes every day. The most appropriate first-line medical management of his symptoms is:
   A Bilateral submandibular gland excision
   B Duct diversion surgery
   C Oral motor exercises
   D Glycopyrronium bromide
   E Botulinum toxin injections

28. A 3-day-old neonate with inspiratory stridor and dyspnoea is noted to have bilateral vocal fold paralysis on flexible nasolaryngoscopy. MRI brain is performed. What is the most commonly found neurological abnormality?
   A Hypoxic-ischaemic encephalopathy

B Choroid plexus cyst
C Arnold-Chiari malformation
D Hydrocephalus
E Superficial siderosis

29. You are reviewing a 1-year-old boy who has been operated on for choanal atresia and your examination reveals a large posterior septal perforation. The airway is patent. What would be your next step in management?
   A Biopsy the mucosa
   B Watchful waiting since it is most likely going to be asymptomatic
   C Counsel the mother, follow up and plan septoplasty in the future
   D Plan to insert a septal button
   E Plan an immediate repair to prevent scar tissue from forming

30. Nasal obstruction secondary to large inferior turbinates is a relatively common problem in children. Regarding surgical procedures for the treatment of enlarged inferior turbinates, which statement is true?
   A Lateralisation/outfracture procedures only offer short-term effect
   B Electrocautery is associated with bleeding, crusting and synechiae formation but has good long-term effect
   C Partial and total resection has better long-term effects than submucous resection
   D Submucous resection is complicated with a significant risk of post-operative anosmia
   E Surgery should be considered first-line once the diagnosis is made

31. For mild OSA and allergic rhinitis in children, intranasal corticosteroids are typically prescribed. Which is true concerning intranasal corticosteroids?
   A 90% of the drug is systemically absorbed
   B Lipophilic drugs like fluticasone propionate have a long elimination time

C Less lipophilic drugs like budesonide have a long elimination time

D Fluticasone propionate is metabolised to fluticasone

E Use of these drugs for over 1 year carry a significant risk of iatrogenic Cushing's syndrome

32. **Tonsillectomies are one of the commonest surgical procedures undertaken in children. The use of a single IV dose of dexamethasone at tonsillectomy:**

A Reduces post-operative bleeding risk

B Reduces post-operative nausea and vomiting

C Is associated with worse post-operative pain

D Is contraindicated in children under 2 years

E Is selectively given for only those at risk of airway obstruction

33. **You are reviewing a 3-week-old neonate and you notice she has a pit in her nasal dorsum. What is the next most appropriate step?**

A MRI scan of the brain

B High-resolution contrasted CT scan of the brain

C Ultrasound of the brain and facial soft tissue

D Referral to neurosurgery and plastic surgery

E List for surgical removal by ENT

34. **Dysphagia is a common presentation in paediatrics. Which of the following is true concerning the protective function of the larynx during swallowing?**

A The epiglottis plays no role in protecting the larynx

B Contraction of the true cords but not the false cords is the main protective mechanism

C Contraction of the false and true vocal cords is the main protective mechanism

D The glottis is closed by adduction of the cuneiforms

E A cough only happens on aspiration of foreign material

35. **The narrowest part of the neonatal airway is the:**

A Supraglottis

B Subglottis

C Post-nasal space

D Glottis

E Carina

36. **A 7-year-old child born 5 weeks premature with a history of prolonged intubation undergoes direct laryngoscopy for noisy breathing. This reveals a 75% subglottic stenosis. What is the grade of subglottic stenosis based on the Cotton-Myer classification?**

A Grade I

B Grade II

C Grade III

D Grade IV

E Grade V

37. **A haemodynamically unstable 14-year-old child is admitted with a post-tonsillectomy bleed necessitating surgery and a blood transfusion. The parents are Jehovah's Witnesses and have refused to give consent. The child also wishes not to be transfused. Which of the following options best represents the appropriate course of action?**

A Contact the Jehovah's Witness liaison committee and monitor the child until they arrive

B Proceed with the transfusion only if the child gives consent

C Do not proceed with the transfusion

D Request a specific issue order

E Proceed with the transfusion because it is in the best interest of the child

38. **A 14-year-old boy presents with a 12-month history of intermittent vertigo. Otoscopic examination reveals normal tympanic membranes. On pneumatic otoscopy he develops a sensation of dizziness and nystagmus is induced. What clinical sign is being elicited?**

A Aquino's sign

B Hitselberger's sign
C Tullio sign
D Hennebert's sign
E Schwartze sign

39. **A 5-year-old boy presents with a 2-month history of chronic nasal obstruction and purulent rhinorrhoea. Flexible nasendoscopy demonstrates a polypoid growth filling the right side of the nose. Biopsy confirms rhabdomyosarcoma. What is the most likely histological subtype?**
   A Alveolar
   B Pleomorphic
   C Undifferentiated sarcoma
   D Anaplastic
   E Embryonal

40. **A 12-year-old boy presents with a worsening of his right-side hearing on the background of bilateral sensorineural hearing loss. He is otherwise fit and well but was recently hit by a car whilst crossing the road on the way home from school. Which condition most likely accounts for his hearing loss?**
   A Usher's syndrome
   B Enlarged vestibular aqueduct
   C Waardenburg syndrome
   D Cogan's syndrome
   E Jervell and Lange-Nielsen

41. **With regard to syndromic hearing loss, which of the following is true?**
   A Pendred's syndrome has autosomal dominant inheritance
   B Jervell and Lange-Nielsen syndrome results from mutations affecting a sodium channel gene
   C In Usher's syndrome Type I, vestibular function is absent
   D Apert syndrome is X-linked
   E Waardenburg syndrome is associated with conductive hearing loss

42. **You are reviewing a 10-year-old boy in clinic who presents with progressive SNHL and worsening vision. You notice from the chart he also has chronic renal**

failure. He tells you that his sister also has the same condition but is less affected. **What is his likely diagnosis?**
   A Goldenhar syndrome
   B Branchio-oto-renal syndrome
   C Pendred syndrome
   D Waardenburg syndrome
   E Alport syndrome

43. **A 5-year-old girl with a history of recurrent respiratory infections presents with increasing nasal obstruction that has not responded to nasal decongestants or steroids. On examination she has bilateral nasal polyps filling both nasal cavities. What is the most appropriate next step?**
   A Skin prick allergy testing
   B CT sinuses
   C Sweat test
   D MRI scan of the sinuses
   E Autoimmune blood panel

44. **A 3-year-old girl is brought to accident and emergency with a low-grade fever, a barking cough and biphasic stridor. What sign on chest radiograph would most likely support the clinical diagnosis?**
   A Steeple sign
   B Double ring sign
   C Halo sign
   D Holman-Miller sign
   E Thumbprint sign

45. **A 3-year-old boy presents with a slowly enlarging painless right submandibular neck lump with progressive violet discolouration of the overlying skin. It has not been responsive to treatment with flucloxacillin. Which of the following should be avoided?**
   A Full surgical excision
   B Clarithromycin +/- rifampicin
   C Culture and sensitivity
   D Incision and drainage
   E None of the above

46. **Shortly after birth a neonate develops respiratory distress, feeding difficulties and abdominal distension. He is**

drooling. What is the most likely anomaly accounting for these symptoms?

A Isolated oesophageal atresia without tracheoesophageal fistula

B Oesophageal atresia with proximal tracheoesophageal fistula

C Oesophageal atresia with distal tracheoesophageal fistula

D Oesophageal atresia with proximal and distal tracheoesophageal fistula

E Isolated tracheoesophageal fistula

47. A diagnosis of Opitz G/BBB is suspected in an infant with ocular hypertelorism and hypospadias presenting with difficulty swallowing and recurrent episodes of pneumonia. What is the gold standard investigation to investigate the associated laryngeal abnormality?

A Modified barium swallow

B Microlaryngobronchoscopy

C Chest X-ray

D Videofluoroscopy

E Flexible nasendoscopy

48. An 18-month-old child presents with a midline nasal dorsal swelling which has recently increased in size. It has been present since birth. Furstenberg's sign is positive. What is the most likely diagnosis?

A Nasal dermoid

B Meningocele

C Nasal glioma

D Dacryocystocele

E Haemangioma

49. A 3-month-old girl presents with inspiratory stridor since birth which is getting worse. She has failure to thrive and has dropped from the fiftieth to the second centile on the paediatric growth chart. Mum reports frequent breaks during breastfeeding. She has a normal cry. Flexible nasendoscopy reveals an omega-shaped epiglottis, shortened aryepiglottic folds and inward collapse of the arytenoids and epiglottis into the laryngeal inlet during inspiration. What is the best management option?

A Regularly monitor weight

B Initiate anti-reflux treatment

C Thicken feeds

D Aryepiglottoplasty

E Tracheostomy

50. A 4-year-old boy presents with severe sore throat, fever, drooling and neck stiffness with a preference for holding his neck in flexion. What is the most likely diagnosis?

A Retropharyngeal abscess

B Peritonsillar abscess

C Epiglottitis

D Tonsillitis

E Inhaled foreign body

51. A previously healthy 15-year-old boy presents with respiratory distress, fever, rigors and neck pain. Symptoms were preceded by a 7-day history of sore throat. He started a course of Amoxicillin 3 days ago. On examination he has swollen exudative tonsils, neck stiffness and tenderness and induration over the angle of the mandible. What is the most likely causative organism?

A *Streptococcus pyogenes*

B *Bacteroides fragilis*

C *Fusobacterium necrophorum*

D *Mycoplasma pneumoniae*

E Epstein-Barr virus

52. You review a newborn baby with acute respiratory distress and cyanosis at rest which is relieved by crying and aggravated by feeding. You are unable to pass a 6Fr suction catheter through either side of the nose. Which of the following is the most appropriate next step?

A Insert McGovern nipple (intraoral airway)

B Administer decongestant, suction the nose and request CT scan

C Insert a nasopharyngeal airway

D Perform flexible nasendoscopy

E Genetic testing for *CHD7* mutations

53. You review a 4-year-old girl with right nasal obstruction and mucoid rhinorrhoea. CT demonstrates posterior nasal narrowing with an obstruction on the right consistent with choanal atresia.

What is the most likely associated
anomaly?
A Michel aplasia
B Hypertelorism
C Thymic aplasia
D Mondini malformation
E Hypoparathyroidism

54. You see a 24-month-old child with
right otalgia and acute onset right
facial nerve palsy. On examination
the child is irritable and pyrexial. A CT
scan reveals no intracranial collection
or coalescent mastoiditis. Otoscopy
reveals a bulging erythematous tympanic membrane. What is the best
management option?
A Commence oral antibiotics
B Admit for IV antibiotics, corticosteroids and aciclovir
C Admit for IV antibiotics and perform
myringotomy and grommet insertion
D Admit for IV antibiotics and perform
cortical mastoidectomy
E Admit and perform mastoidectomy
and facial nerve decompression

55. You review a child with odynophagia, fever and trismus. You are unable
to examine the child because he
becomes too distressed. What is the
next most appropriate step?
A Perform a full blood count and measure CRP
B List for examination under
anaesthetic
C Perform CT scan of the neck with
contrast
D Perform non-contrast CT scan
E Perform transoral ultrasound

56. You are reviewing an 8-year-old girl
who has had 3 episodes of acute left-
sided suppurative thyroiditis. What
is the most likely branchial system
anomaly?
A First branchial cleft
B Second branchial cleft
C Third branchial cleft
D Third branchial pouch
E Third branchial arch

57. A 2-year-old boy is brought to the ED by
his mother with reports of choking and
coughing. Earlier in the day the boy's
brother gave him some cashew nuts.
Observations are stable and there is no
evidence of respiratory distress; however, whilst you are examining him you
notice that he has an intermittent cough.
His mother tells you he has not been
unwell lately and this is a new cough.
A chest X-ray shows no abnormality.
Examination of the chest is unremarkable. What is the most appropriate next
action?
A Repeat chest X-ray
B MRI thorax
C CT thorax
D Rigid bronchoscopy
E Flexible laryngoscopy

58. You are called at 2 a.m. to ED to review
a 3-year-old boy who has been brought
in by his mother who found the child
coughing in his bed. There is a suspicion that a bead is missing from a
necklace. On examination, the child
appears comfortable and all observations are stable. Auscultation of the
chest reveals an inspiratory wheeze
and an X-ray reveals a foreign body
in the right main bronchus. What is the
most appropriate next action?
A Repeat chest X-ray
B Flexible nasendoscopy
C Flexible bronchoscopy
D Emergency rigid bronchoscopy
E List for rigid bronchoscopy as the first
case in the morning

59. You are in a paediatric ENT outpatient
clinic and reviewing an 18-month-
old girl who has been diagnosed
with a subglottic haemangioma. You
note from the case notes that medical therapy has been recommended.
Which investigation would be the most
appropriate next step?
A Full blood count
B Echocardiogram
C Electrocardiogram

D CT chest
E Lung function test

60. **A 10-year-old boy presents to the ED with a 1-week history of odynophagia, fever and reduced neck movements. Antibiotics have not yet been started. On examination he has torticollis and intraoral examination is normal apart from evidence of oropharyngeal mucus. There is no respiratory distress and apart from fever the observations are normal. A CT neck with contrast reveals a 0.8 x 0.9 cm retropharyngeal collection suggestive of abscess. What is the next most appropriate step?**
   A Emergency per oral incision and drainage under general anaesthesia
   B Emergency transcervical incision and drainage under general anaesthesia
   C Oral antibiotics with clinic review in 3 days
   D Admit for IV antibiotics
   E Recommend intubation by paediatric anaesthesia

61. **Children can decompensate precipitously. The narrowest location in the airway is:**
   A Adult: glottis; Child: subglottis
   B Adult: subglottis; Child: glottis
   C Adult: supraglottis; Child: subglottis
   D Adult: subglottis; Child: supraglottis
   E Adult: trachea; Child: subglottis

62. **A 3-year-old child is admitted with stridor which responds to nebulised adrenaline. According to Poiseuille's law (the Hagen–Poiseuille equation), a 50% reduction in the radius of the airway results in:**
   A 50% increase in resistance to airflow
   B 4-fold increase in resistance to airflow
   C 8-fold increase in resistance to airflow
   D 25% increase in resistance to airflow
   E 16-fold increase in resistance to airflow

63. **You are reviewing a 3-year-old boy in clinic. He was 6 weeks premature and required intubation on the neonatal unit. He has had frequent respiratory tract infections throughout his life. With these episodes his mother has noticed his breathing becomes noisy. The most common cause of subglottic stenosis is:**
   A Congenital
   B Inhalational burns
   C Meconium aspiration
   D Acquired subglottic stenosis
   E Caustic ingestion

64. **Which of the following presentations is most likely associated with subglottic stenosis?**
   A Inspiratory stridor with severe dysphonia
   B Biphasic or inspiratory stridor with mild or no voice change
   C Expiratory stridor with hoarseness
   D Tachypnoea and subcostal retractions
   E No stridor with severe dysphonia

65. **Cardiac surgery is a common cause for vocal cord palsy in children. Which of the following is true concerning the innervation of the larynx?**
   A The left recurrent laryngeal nerve arises from the vagus to the left of the arch of the aorta. It curves inferior to the aortic arch and ascends in the groove between the trachea and the oesophagus. This extensive course is the reason it is more commonly injured.
   B The right recurrent laryngeal nerve arises from the vagus to the right of the arch of the aorta. It curves inferior to the aortic arch and ascends in the groove between the trachea and the oesophagus. This extensive course is the reason it is more commonly injured.
   C The recurrent laryngeal nerve supplies the cricothyroid muscle
   D The superior laryngeal nerve supplies the vocalis muscle
   E The recurrent laryngeal nerve supplies sensation to the supraglottis

66. **During a microlaryngoscopy and bronchoscopy (MLB) you are assessing the airway of a 1-year-old boy who had presented with recurrent respiratory**

infections and intermittent stridor. When sizing the airway, if the endotracheal tube (ETT) has a leak at pressures of <5–10 cm H20:

A This confirms the ETT is the correct size
B A smaller ETT should be used
C A cuffed ETT should be used
D An uncuffed ETT should be used
E A larger ETT should be used

67. **You decide to perform an endoscopic dilation of a subglottic stenosis in a 3-year-old boy. The best candidate for an endoscopic balloon dilatation is:**
A Thick, mature stenosis
B Circumferential stenosis
C Thin web-like stenosis
D Grade 1 stenosis
E Grade 1 and 2 stenosis

68. **You are about to perform microlaryngoscopy and bronchoscopy (MLB) on a 1-year-old to investigate recurrent stridor. Regarding muscle paralysis in MLB, which statement is most appropriate?**
A Muscle paralysis is favoured to stop any patient movements
B Muscle paralysis is usually not required
C Muscle paralysis is contraindicated
D Muscle paralysis is favoured to allow spontaneous ventilation
E Muscle paralysis is not utilised, so as to allow for spontaneous ventilation

69. **A child with a tracheostomy in situ for subglottic stenosis wishes to be decannulated. Which of the following is a contraindication to single-stage laryngotracheal reconstruction?**
A Central/obstructive sleep apnoea precluding decannulation
B Good voice at baseline
C Body weight of 11 kg
D On treatment with proton pump inhibitor
E On double treatment for gastro-oesophageal reflux

70. **Under which of the following circumstances is a laryngeal keel most useful?**
A Anterior glottic stenosis
B Posterior glottic stenosis
C Congenital subglottic stenosis
D Acquired subglottic stenosis
E Supraglottic stenosis

71. **Congenital subglottic stenosis:**
A Usually presents at 1 week after birth
B Usually presents at 1 month after birth
C Results from incomplete recanalisation of the laryngotracheal tube during the third month of gestation
D Results from incomplete recanalisation of the laryngotracheal tube during the sixth month of gestation
E Can be caused by meconium aspiration

72. **Which of the following is not considered one of the advantages of awake flexible laryngoscopy?**
A Can assess vocal fold mobility
B Can effectively/thoroughly assess the subglottis
C Can assess dynamic supraglottic pathology
D Can be done on awake children of any age
E Can be done bedside or in a clinic setting

73. **A tracheostomy is most likely to be required under which circumstance?**
A Anterior and posterior glottic stenosis
B Anterior and posterior subglottic stenosis
C Salvage after failure of laryngotracheal reconstruction
D Myer-Cotton grade 3 stenosis
E Firm grade 1 Myer-Cotton stenosis

74. **Which is considered the strongest graft for laryngotracheal reconstruction?**
A Auricular cartilage
B Tragal cartilage
C Thyroid alar cartilage
D Nasal septal cartilage
E Costal cartilage

75. **What does single-stage laryngotracheal reconstruction imply?**
A The procedure is definitive and one is confident a revision is not necessary

B Costal cartilage grafting is used

C A tracheostomy is used to 'cover' the procedure

D A tracheostomy is either removed during reconstruction (if present pre-operatively), or not placed

E The patient is extubated immediately after the reconstruction

76. **You are performing an adenoidectomy on a 5-year-old boy with OSA. Your examination in theatre reveals a submu-cous cleft. How should you proceed?**

A Complete a full adenoidectomy

B Perform an inferior adenoidectomy

C Perform a superior adenoidectomy

D Perform a shallow adenoidectomy

E Abandon the procedure and offer only medical treatment

77. **Which of the following is true of Eustachian tube dysfunction (ETD) in children with cleft lip/palate?**

A ETD in children with cleft lip results from the abnormal insertion of the levator and tensor veli palatini

B Ear tubes are placed by 3 months of age

C ETD in children with cleft palate results from the abnormal insertion of the levator and tensor veli palatini

D ETD in children with cleft lip and alveolus results from the abnormal insertion of the levator and tensor veli palatini

E Ear tubes are placed by 6 months of age

78. **Which of the following nipples is best suited for feeding infants with cleft lip/palate?**

A Haberman nipple

B Level 1 nipple

C Ultrapremie nipple

D Preemie nipple

E McGovern nipple

79. **A 5-year-old boy has a diagnosis of recurrent respiratory papillomatosis and has required 5 surgical debulkings this**

year. **Which medication would be the most appropriate next step?**

A Cidofovir

B Interferon beta

C Bevacizumab

D Tacrolimus

E Mitomycin C

80. **You are seeing an 11-year-old girl in clinic who has been referred in for a hoarse voice for the last year. There are no other airway symptoms. Her mother tells you she is a keen singer. She becomes very distressed when you suggest flexible nasendoscopy. The next most appropriate step is:**

A Reassure and discharge

B CT neck with contrast

C List for microlaryngoscopy and bronchoscopy

D Referral for speech therapy

E MRI neck with contrast

81. **You are reviewing a 9-year-old boy with cerebral palsy and neurodevelopmental delay. He has a long-term tracheos-tomy for airway protection. His parents have noticed that his voice has become rougher over the last 6 months. The most likely cause is:**

A Tracheostomy tube misplaced

B Tracheostomy tube too small

C Suprastomal granulation

D Distal tracheal granulation

E Laryngeal nodules

82. **You are reviewing a 3-year-old boy in clinic. His mother is concerned about his prominent ears. She was teased at school about her own ears and is worried about her child starting school in the next year. Examination reveals bilateral prominau-ris. The next most appropriate step is:**

A Reassure and follow up in a year

B List for bilateral otoplasty

C Recommend splinting

D Recommend counselling for the mother and child

E Reassure, discharge and suggest re-referral after age 5 as required

83. **You are called to the ED to review a 5-year-old girl with a lip laceration. The ED doctor suspects that this may be a non-accidental injury. What is the next most appropriate step?**
   A Proceed with suturing the lip laceration in the ED
   B Consult the plastic surgery team for repair in theatre
   C Explain your suspicions to the parent and perform a full examination to look for other injuries
   D Contact the paediatric team to report the suspicion of non-accidental injury
   E Contact social services to report the suspicion of non-accidental injury

84. **A 4-year-old boy presents with an enlarging left level 2 neck mass over the last 6 months. He has already had 2 courses of antibiotics from his GP. Last month an incision and drainage was performed for a suspected neck abscess at another hospital. Currently the skin over the mass has a violaceous quality with small areas of tissue breakdown. Surgical excision is performed. What is the characteristic histopathology finding in this condition?**
   A Caseating granulomas with central necrosis and multinucleated giant cells
   B Orphan Annie nuclei
   C Non-caseating granulomas without necrosis
   D Non-granulomatous inflammation with vasculitis
   E Non-granulomatous inflammation with fat necrosis

85. **You are asked to review a 6-year-old girl who has been referred because she has a profound hearing impairment and she is struggling with her speech development. Her mother tells you she has recently started to wear glasses because her vision has been getting worse. She was slow to meet her motor developmental milestones and has problems with her balance. The most likely diagnosis is:**
   A Usher syndrome
   B Alport syndrome
   C CHARGE syndrome
   D Apert syndrome
   E Stickler syndrome

86. **You are called urgently to paediatric resus to assess a 12-year-old boy who fell off his skateboard 6 hours ago, hitting his neck against a metal railing. He has a mild inspiratory stridor with O2 saturations of 100% on 2 L. His observations are stable and he has no voice change. There is no evidence of surgical emphysema. Which of these options is the most appropriate step?**
   A Increase O2 to 4L
   B Observe in ED majors
   C Transfer to paediatric ITU
   D Secure airway in ED via orotracheal intubation
   E Transfer to theatre to secure airway

87. **A 5-year-old boy is bitten on the nose by a stray dog in a local park. He was staying with his biological father at the time of the incident but he usually lives with his mother because the parents have recently divorced. The decision is made that this needs to be cleaned and sutured in theatre. Which of these options is the most appropriate step?**
   A No consent is necessary since the child can be treated in his best interests
   B His mother should be contacted for consent
   C His father may give consent
   D The local authority should be contacted to provide consent
   E The hospital legal team should be contacted for advice before any treatment can be given

88. **You are reviewing a 4-year-old boy who has unilateral grade 3 microtia. His parents are interested in surgical options. How early is microtia reconstruction advised?**
   A 5–7 years

B   As soon as is possible
C   6–8 years
D   8–10 years
E   Never before 18 years

89. **Which of the following options is a contraindication for cochlear implantation in children?**
    A   Mondini deformity
    B   Enlarged vestibular aqueduct
    C   Hypoplastic cochlear nerve
    D   Absent cochlear nerve
    E   A and D

90. **What is the most common cause of congenital tracheal stenosis?**
    A   CMV-related in-utero infection
    B   Syphilis-related in-utero infection
    C   Bronchus suis
    D   Complete tracheal rings
    E   Toxoplasma-related in-utero infection

91. **You are reviewing a 7-year-old girl with trisomy 21 in clinic. Her parents are concerned about her noisy breathing at night. Of the following options, which anatomical factor primarily accounts for her symptoms?**
    A   Laryngomalacia
    B   Narrow nasopharynx
    C   Muscle hypotonia
    D   Midface and mandibular hypoplasia
    E   All of the above

92. **In the case of OSA refractory to adenotonsillectomy in a child with trisomy 21, the most common site of residual obstruction is:**
    A   Supraglottis
    B   Gottis
    C   Nasopharynx
    D   Base of tongue
    E   Pharynx

93. **You are reviewing a 10-year-old girl with trisomy 21 and OSA in clinic. She has previously had an adenoidectomy and base-of-tongue reduction but is still having significant OSA. Her parents have heard about selective hypoglossal nerve stimulation and wish to**

discuss this further. Its mechanism of action is:
    A   Activation of the key muscles of the upper airway to ensure the airway remains open
    B   Activation of the key muscles of the larynx to ensure the airway remains open
    C   Deactivation of the key contracted muscles of the upper airway to ensure the airway remains open
    D   Deactivation the key contracted muscles of the larynx to ensure the airway remains open
    E   A and D

94. **On the effect of age/maturation on auditory nerve and brainstem evoked potentials (ABEP), which of the following is true?**
    A   After 26 weeks, components II, IV and VI are well defined
    B   At birth, latencies are similar to adults
    C   In premature neonates, ABEPs are not detectable before 26 weeks gestational age
    D   Interpeak latency differences lengthen with maturation
    E   Wave V latency is shortened in extremely premature infants

95. **You are called to the ED to assess a 7-year-old boy weighing 20 kg who has been readmitted with a post-tonsillectomy bleed. On assessment the child is not actively bleeding. The heart rate is 102 beats per minute and the blood pressure is 110/90 mmHg. What is the minimum volume of blood loss that would trigger a tachycardia in this child?**
    A   125 ml
    B   225 ml
    C   325 ml
    D   425 ml
    E   500 ml

96. **An 18-month-old boy born at 35 weeks gestation via spontaneous vaginal delivery undergoes**

microlaryngoscopy and bronchoscopy due to a history of stridor and recurrent pneumonia. Partial cricoid cleft remaining above the cricoid lamina is noted. According to the Benjamin Inglis classification, what type of cleft is this?

A Type 0
B Type I
C Type II
D Type III
E Type IV

97. You see a 5-year-old boy in clinic with a 6-week history of right-sided post grommet mucoid otorrhoea. He has not been practising strict water precautions. What is the most appropriate next step in management?

A Microsuction the ear
B Advise strict water precautions
C Microsuction the ear and prescribe a course of ciprofloxacin ear drops
D Microsuction the ear and prescribe an oral course of Amoxicillin
E Microsuction the ear and organise for the patient to have the grommet removed

98. With regard to Usher syndrome, which of the following is true?

A There are 5 types
B It is the most common cause of deafblindness
C Vestibular function is normal in Type I

D It is the most common cause of autosomal dominant syndromic hearing loss
E It results from mutations affecting a potassium channel gene

99. You see a 5-year-old girl with a history of dysphonia and shortness of breath. The child undergoes repeat microlaryngoscopy and bronchoscopy and biopsy which demonstrates further 'grape like' lesions in the larynx and new distal tracheal disease. Biopsy and HPV typing identifies HPV 11. What further investigation should be performed?

A CT chest
B CT neck
C MRI neck
D MRI chest
E Barium swallow

100. You review a 5-month-old child in clinic. She has developed a 4 cm mass in the right parotid region. Her mother tells you that it started as a peanut-sized lump about 3 months ago. On examination the mass is soft and non-fluctuant and there is evidence of skin telangiectasia over the surface. The most likely diagnosis is:

A Pleomorphic adenoma
B Acute parotitis
C Mucoepidermoid carcinoma
D Parotid gland haemangioma
E First branchial arch anomaly

PAEDIATRICS

1. **Answer C**

   Intracranial infections in children are rare but have the potential to cause significant neurological sequelae. Focal intracranial infections can be classified based on their anatomical location: epidural abscess, subdural empyema and brain abscess. A brain abscess is an encapsulated focal area of brain necrosis within the brain parenchyma resulting from an infectious or traumatic process. Brain abscesses begin as areas of cerebritis and progress to encapsulated pus within 2 weeks. An epidural abscess is a collection of pus between the dura mater and the skull. A subdural empyema is a collection of pus between the dura mater and arachnoid mater. A subdural empyema appears crescentic in shape compared to epidural abscesses that are lentiform (lens-shaped). A subdural empyema crosses cranial sutures whereas epidural abscesses are contained by the sutures.

   Otitis media, mastoiditis, dental and sinus infections cause intracranial infection via direct local spread. Most cases present with non-specific signs resulting in a delay in diagnosis. The classic triad of headache, fever and focal neurologic deficit is rarely seen. Non-specific symptoms such as headache, nausea, vomiting and fevers present early in the development of an intracranial infection. Mental status change, papilledema and seizures result from raised intracranial pressure; however, irritability is the most common first sign of intracranial infection in infants. It is critical that clinicians be aware that broad non-specific symptoms, such as irritability, in the context of infection, should raise suspicion of something more serious in a child.

2. **Answer B**

   Pendred syndrome is an autosomal recessive genetic disorder consisting of bilateral sensorineural hearing loss and goitre (euthyroid or hypothyroid). It is the most common syndromic form of hearing loss. The condition results from mutations in the *PDS* gene (coding for the SLC26A4 protein). Mutations in this gene are also associated with enlarged vestibular aqueduct syndrome. A mixed hearing loss may result from the third window effect of the inner ear malformation. In a perchlorate discharge test iodide (I123) is given orally followed an hour later by 600 mg perchlorate intravenously. Perchlorate displaces non-organified iodide from the thyroid. In Pendred there is a defect in iodine organification. An abnormal result is defined as a release of >20% of the radioactive iodide taken up by the thyroid gland.

3. **Answer B**

   Neonates are obligate nasal breathers; hence even a small reduction in the nasal airway can result in significant respiratory distress. Neonatal rhinitis is the most common cause of nasal obstruction in the neonate. Neonatal rhinitis describes inflammation of the sinonasal mucosa. GORD and nasopharyngeal milk regurgitation are common causes of neonatal rhinitis. Topical intranasal steroids (1 week) or decongestants such as phenylephrine (0.125%), oxymetazoline (0.025%) (3 days) or xylometazoline (0.05% Otrivine, 5 days, note that this is an off-licence use in children <1 year the UK) are effective treatments.

4. **Answer E**

   The branchial arch system develops in the fourth week of gestation and consists of six paired arches. Each has a cartilage component, a muscle component and an associated cranial nerve and artery. The trigeminal nerve is associated with the first branchial arch supplying motor supply to the muscles of mastication and muscles of the first arch including anterior digastric, tensor veli palatini, tensor tympani and mylohyoid. Sensory supply is to the face via the ophthalmic, maxillary and mandibular branches. The first branchial arch is also the origin for the internal maxillary artery, external carotid artery, mandible (rudiment) and the malleus and incus from Meckel's cartilage. The facial nerve, although in anatomical proximity to the cyst and hence the importance of using a facial nerve monitor, is derived from the second branchial arch. In this case the location of the cyst is suggestive of a first branchial cleft cyst. First branchial cleft cysts compose less than 1% of branchial anomalies. These are divided into type 1 and 2 (Work classification). Type 1 cysts appear as duplication of the external auditory canal and contain epidermoid elements without cartilage and remain lateral to the facial nerve. Type 2 cysts contain ectoderm and mesoderm and pass either medial or lateral to the facial nerve and run from the floor of the ear canal into the neck. USS is an acceptable diagnostic tool although increasingly MRI evaluation of soft tissues is preferred.

5. **Answer D**

    Solitary median maxillary incisor syndrome is a developmental disorder consisting of multiple midline abnormalities. Additional to the central megaincisor, abnormalities include congenital nasal malformations (choanal atresia, congenital pyriform aperture stenosis). Holoprosencephaly (HPE) is a serious associated anomaly in which the embryonic forebrain does not develop two separate hemispheres. Based on the severity of the defect HPE is classified into three subtypes of reducing severity: alobar, semilobar and lobar. Eighty percent of HPE are associated with facial abnormalities with cyclopia and proboscis formation associated with the severe forms and central megaincisor and nasal defects associated with the milder forms of HPE.

6. **Answer B**

    Sandifer syndrome (SS) is a form of non-epileptic paroxysmal dystonia causing spasms of the head, neck and back but with sparing of the limbs. SS is commonly associated with gastroesophageal reflux disease (GORD). Typically, the dystonic events occur shortly after feeding with improvement in between feeds. If there are features more consistent with epileptic seizures (e.g. occurring during sleep, loss of consciousness) then an evaluation by a paediatric neurologist is warranted. SS responds to treatment of the underlying GORD either by non-pharmacological methods (e.g. thickening feeds, reducing feeding volumes) or pharmacological treatments (proton pump inhibitors and anti-reflux medications). Infantile colic, which is typically synonymous with GORD, may present similarly, but the presence of neck spasms is more suggestive of SS.

7. **Answer A**

    Craniosynostosis is a condition in which one or more of the fibrous sutures in an infant skull prematurely ossifies and fuses. The skull will then compensate by growing parallel to the closed suture (since growth perpendicular to the closed suture is not possible). Craniosynostosis is part of a syndrome in 15–40% of cases (e.g. Apert, Crouzon, Muenke syndrome); the remainder of cases occur in isolation. Depending on the level of brain compression there may be associated visual and neurodevelopmental impairment. Syndromic forms occur in the context of other systemic features, e.g. digital abnormalities in Apert syndrome. The syndromic forms of craniosynostosis have a high risk of developing obstructive sleep apnoea.

Craniosynostosis subtypes and the affected suture are listed here:

Scaphocephaly – sagittal suture (narrow skull, most common subtype)

Plagiocephaly – anterior plagiocephaly (unilateral coronal synostosis, skew head), posterior plagiocephaly (unilateral synostosis, skew head)

Brachycephaly – coronal suture (short head)

Kleeblattschaedel – sagittal, coronal and lambdoid sutures (cloverleaf skull, bulging of cranial contents)

Trigonocephaly – metopic suture (triangular forehead)

8. **Answer C**

DiGeorge syndrome (22q11.2 deletion syndrome, microdeletion encompassing 30–50 genes, including *TBX1* and *DGCR8*, on long arm of chromosome 22) is usually detected using fluorescence in situ hybridisation (FISH) or quantitative polymerase chain reaction (qPCR) to detect the microdeletion. Ninety per cent of cases are caused by a de novo mutation. The clinical presentation is summarised by the acronym CATCH-22—**C**ardiac abnormalities (tetralogy of Fallot, truncus arteriosus, interrupted aortic arch), **A**bnormal facies (including velopharyngeal insufficiency), **T**hymic aplasia (deficiency in T cell maturation leading to immunodeficiency, **C**left palate, **H**ypoparathyroidism (hypocalcaemia). Treatment is symptomatic, addressing each of the associated features individually.

9. **Answer C**

A 2% solution of lignocaine contains 20 mg/ml lignocaine. The maximum safe dose of lignocaine with adrenaline is 7 mg/kg. Therefore, the maximum dose for a 15 kg child is 105 mg (7 mg/kg x 15 kg). The maximum safe volume is therefore 5.25 ml (105 mg/20 mg/ml).

10. **Answer A**

In this scenario CT imaging of the temporal bone and brain is indicated. Contrast is required to assess for intracranial abscess and dural sinus thrombosis. An MRI brain with contrast would be useful for intracranial complications but is limited in its delineation of the bony anatomy that is useful in surgical planning. Additionally, CT scanning in a 3-year-old child may require general anaesthesia; hence IV access is the most appropriate first stage in management.

11. **Answer D**

Vascular compression of the trachea is a rare but important cause of chronic respiratory disease in childhood. The aberrant innominate artery is the most common vascular sling, a congenital malformation resulting from the abnormal development of the great vessels. Vascular rings can be complete or incomplete (sling) and include the double aortic arch (most common), pulmonary sling and the aberrant right subclavian artery. The pattern of indentation on videofluoroscopy, bronchoscopy, air tracheogram and the use of CT angiogram can be used in diagnosis. The aberrant innominate artery demonstrates anterior-only tracheal indentation at LTB.

12. **Answer A**

High volume epistaxis in an adolescent boy is suggestive of juvenile nasopharyngeal angiofibroma (JNA) a rare, highly vascular tumour that arises in the posterior nasal cavity almost exclusively in adolescent boys. Although benign it displays aggressive behaviour invading local structures. It arises from the sphenopalatine foramen and posterior nasal cavity. It may extend into the nasal cavity, nasopharynx and ptery-gopalatine fossa. More extensive disease can spread to the sphenoid, ethmoid and maxillary sinuses, the orbit and intracranially. Blood supply is via the internal maxillary artery, a branch of the external carotid artery but there may be recruitment of vessels from the internal carotid including the ophthalmic and Vidian artery. The most appropriate first step in investigating the cause of this child's epistaxis is a contrast-enhanced CT sinuses. This typically reveals a heterodense mass centred on the sphenopalatine foramen that avidly enhances. Characteristic anterior bowing of the posterior maxillary wall due to the tumour is known as the Holman-Miller sign. MRI is useful adjunct and provides superior detection of intracranial extension. MRI reveals a T1 hypodense, T2 intermediate lesion with avid enhancement and flow voids with contrast enhancement. Biopsy without imaging is not recommended due to the risk of haemorrhage. Surgical resection is the mainstay of treatment and pre-operative embolisation is recommended although there is evidence that this may increase the risk of residual disease.

13. Answer A

In this situation the child has a potentially time-critical and life-threatening medical condition. Although the concerns regarding legal guardianship are pertinent, the primary focus should be on the health of the child. In the UK healthcare providers are permitted to provide emergency care to minors in lieu of parental consent if the child's health is at risk. This is known as 'implied consent' for emergency treatment. In this case the first action should be to attempt to contact the child's mother as her legal guardian to establish consent. However, if this is not possible it may be warranted to proceed in draining the neck abscess without consent. In this case one should document that this is a multi-consultant decision (paediatrician/ENT/anaesthetist) taken in the child's best interest. Additionally, consultation with the hospital's legal or ethics team after the immediate medical needs are addressed is recommended.

14. Answer B

PRS consists of a wide U-shaped cleft palate, micrognathia (small mandible) and glossoptosis (downward displaced/retracted tongue, rather than macroglossia). PRS is not a syndrome but a sequence of events resulting from a specific developmental abnormality (mandibular hypoplasia). PRS may occur in isolation or as part of a syndrome, e.g. Stickler syndrome, DiGeorge syndrome, Patau syndrome. It has been suggested that abnormal neck flexion causes mechanical restriction of mandibular growth in utero resulting in restricted room for tongue growth which becomes downwardly displaced and impedes the closure of the palatal shelves leading to cleft palate formation. There is no singular gene abnormality responsible for PRS although mutations in *SOX9*, *KCNJ2* and *GAD1* have been implicated. Airway obstruction results from oropharyngeal and hypopharyngeal obstruction rather than subglottic stenosis. Management focuses on the airway and feeding issues, whilst optimising growth and nutrition.

15. Answer C

Given the clinical history, the most likely diagnosis is tonsillitis. Most commonly these are viral in origin (rhinovirus, parainfluenza, adenovirus, Epstein-Barr virus). The most common bacterial cause of tonsillitis in *Streptococcus pyogenes*.

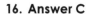

16. **Answer C**

    Many cleaning products are alkalis that are more destructive to tissue since they cause liquefactive necrosis in contrast to acidic solutions which cause coagulative necrosis (which reduces tissue penetration). Initial management consists of prevention of vomiting and aspiration. Neutralisation agents are not recommended due to the exothermic reaction generated on neutralisation. Airway protection is paramount and if there are concerns, endotracheal intubation or tracheostomy should be undertaken. The key role for ENT in this scenario is airway protection. Referral to the paediatric/gastroenterology team is recommended and OGD allows direct visualisation of the oesophagus. In this case, it is crucial for assessing the degree of oesophageal injury. CT imaging is generally not a first-line investigation to assess oesophageal injury caused by toxic ingestions. However, it may be used later to assess for extra-oesophageal complications.

17. **Answer C**

    Surgical drainage, either via endoscopic or external (Lynch-Howarth) approach, of subperiosteal or orbital abscess (Group 3 or 4 in the Chandler classification) is indicated for larger, non-medial collections, significant proptosis, concerns about visual compromise and restricted eye movements. However, small collections, typically no more than 10 mm in diameter, can be managed with a trial of IV antibiotics. An MRI sinuses and brain should be considered if there are concerns of intracranial infection, e.g. meningitis, reduced GCS, suspicion of dural sinus thrombosis.

18. **Answer B**

    For septal abscesses, incision and drainage under general anaesthesia is the preferred approach given that there is a risk of central spread of infection from the danger area of the face into the cavernous sinus. It is likely there has already been cartilage necrosis at this point which may cause septal perforation or saddle nose deformity needing reconstruction in the future. Drainage under local anaesthetic may be challenging and is unlikely to be tolerated by a young child. Needle aspiration is generally unsatisfactory and often leads to re-accumulation of the abscess. Intranasal packing and IV antibiotics are ancillary to incision and drainage but should not be used as a sole treatment.

19. **Answer C**

    The most likely diagnosis is a facial infantile haemangioma. Up to 50% of children with subglottic haemangioma will also have facial haemangiomas, most often in the 'beard' distribution. Glut-1 expression is specific to haemangiomas and can aid diagnosis. A negative Glut-1 expression makes an infantile haemangioma unlikely. A positive Glut-1 excludes a vascular malformation and is suggestive of infantile haemangioma but may also be positive in other lesions such as angiosarcoma, so the test should not be used in isolation. Airway endoscopy is not warranted based solely on the finding of a facial haemangioma, however if there are signs or symptoms of airway compromise then further evaluation is recommended. Observation is recommended if there has been no rapid increase in size, bleeding, ulceration or any signs of airway or functional compromise. Propranolol is an appropriate medical management of infantile subglottic haemangiomas.

20. **Answer C**

    The 'double ring sign' suggests that the foreign body is likely to be a button battery. If a button battery becomes lodged in the oesophagus, an electrical current is generated between the positive and negative poles. Additionally, released hydroxide ions can cause an alkaline injury. Significant injury including oesophageal perforation, stricture and erosion into adjacent critical structures of the mediastinum can occur within hours. The risk of potentially fatal aorto-oesophageal fistula is highest in children under 5, with batteries over 20 mm in diameter and impaction at the level of the aortic arch. Symptoms in young children include gagging, poor feeding, drooling and irritability. In this case, emergent rigid endoscopic removal under general anaesthetic is the most appropriate treatment.

21. **Answer A**

    Infantile subglottic haemangiomas are the most prevalent benign tumours of infancy and may occur as isolated lesions or as part of a segmental haemangioma syndrome such as PHACES (**P**osterior fossa malformations, **H**aemangioma of the cervicofacial region, **A**rterial anomalies, **C**ardiac anomalies, **E**ye anomalies and **S**ternal or abdominal clefting). Typically, they grow rapidly in the first three months of life with the growth phase lasting from 6 to 10 months before beginning to involute. Fifty per cent of these lesions will self-regress by the age of 5. Treatment options include medical (propranolol or steroids) or surgery in medically resistant cases, although surgery has been associated with subglottic stenosis. Commencement of propranolol therapy requires a pre-treatment work up including ECG, blood tests (FBC, U&E, LFT, glucose, TFT) and possibly an ECHO. After appropriate work-up, propranolol is the recommended first-line treatment of infantile subglottic haemangiomas.

22. **Answer B**

    If there is no concern for respiratory distress or any evidence of aspiration (usually judged by a speech and language therapist review +/- a videofluoroscopic swallow study or a flexible endoscopic evaluation of swallowing [FEES]) then there is no indication to proceed to surgical treatment. A period of observation is recommended since spontaneous recovery may occur.

23. **Answer B**

    Laryngeal reinnervation can restore the connection of motor neurons with denervated laryngeal muscles. Neurorrhaphy of the ansa cervicalis to the recurrent laryngeal nerve is often selected for laryngeal reinnervation procedures due to its proximity and availability of suitable nerve fibres for grafting.

24. **Answer C**

    Congenital aural atresia occurs in approximately 1 in 10,000 newborns. It is commonly unilateral, associated with developmental abnormalities of the pinna and may be associated with a syndrome or occur in isolation. The Jahrsdoerfer grading system (Table 3.1) is based on radiological findings and can be used as a prognostic indicator for the success of atresiaplasty (in terms of the post-operative hearing result).

    A score of 10 would be an ideal surgical candidate, a score of 7 would indicate a good candidate and a score under 6 would be a poor surgical candidate. In patients for whom atresiaplasty is not indicated, a bone conduction hearing device may be a useful hearing aid option, e.g. cochlear OSIA or BAHA. This patient would score 5 (microtia, disrupted IM, malformed stapes, sclerotic mastoid) and hence would be a poor candidate for atresiaplasty.

Table 3.1 Jahrsdoerfer Grading Scale

Temporal bone parameter	Score
Stapes present	2
Oval window normal	1
Round window normal	1
Incudo-stapedial connection normal	1
Aerated middle ear cleft	1
Pneumatised mastoid	1
Normal course of facial nerve	1
Malleo-incudal complex normal	1
Normal appearance of external ear	1
Max score	10
Atresia surgery recommended	>7

25. Answer D

It has been reported that 2% of children with unilateral tonsillar enlargement have an underlying tonsillar malignancy. The most common malignancy in these cases is non-Hodgkin's lymphoma. Significant red flags include significant asymmetry (e.g. 2-point difference on the Brodsky scale), enlargement over 3–12 weeks, B symptoms and the presence of cervical lymph nodes. Asymmetric tonsils are common and without other red flag symptoms a period of observation is recommended. Choking on food in a seven-year-old is, however, uncommon and increasingly tonsillectomy is being used to help solid food dysphagia and reduce the risk of potentially life-threatening choking in children.

26. Answer A

The daily maintenance fluid requirements for a child are as follows (this does not apply to neonates 0–28 days after full-term delivery date):

For infants 3.5 to 10 kg – 100 mL/kg.

For children 11–20 kg – 1000 mL + 50 mL/kg for every kg over 10.

For children >20 kg – 1500 mL + 20 mL/kg for every kg over 20, up to a maximum of 2400 mL daily.

Hence for this child the daily maintenance rate is 1500 ml (1000 ml + 10 x 50 ml).

27. Answer D

Drooling is the unintentional loss of saliva from the oral cavity and is a normal phenomenon in many children prior to the development of oral neuromuscular control at age 18–24 months. It is considered abnormal if it persists beyond age 4. Up to 30% of children with cerebral palsy have problematic drooling due to poor neuromuscular control. Drooling is managed in a stepwise fashion depending on the severity, underlying cause and response to prior interventions. There are non-surgical (e.g. SLT assessment/oromotor therapy and medical therapy) and surgical options (including submandibular duct diversion and excision of the submandibular glands). Anticholinergic medication including glycopyrronium bromide (40–100 mcg per kg tds, max 2 mg per dose) and hyoscine hydrobromide (half patch every 72 hours) are first-line medical options. However, adverse effects include dry mouth, thick secretions, urinary retention and constipation.

28. Answer C

Congenital vocal fold paralysis is the second most common cause of stridor in infants. It can be unilateral or bilateral. The most common aetiology is idiopathic. Otherwise, congenital causes include neurological anomalies (e.g. Arnold-Chiari malformation and meningomyelocele) and acquired causes include birth trauma and iatrogenic injury (e.g. cardiac surgery, thyroidectomy, intubation injury). Microlaryngoscopy/bronchoscopy is important to rule out other airway pathologies and to differentiate paralysis from vocal fold fixation by palpation of the cricoarytenoid joint. MRI brain, neck and chest (entire length of the recurrent laryngeal nerve) is important to identify central nervous system (CNS) pathology. Most congenital vocal fold paralysis spontaneously improves in 1 year, although temporary tracheostomy may be required to maintain a safe airway in bilateral cases.

29. Answer B

Posterior septal perforations are usually asymptomatic and, on counselling the family, can be observed. Biopsy of the mucosa to rule out infectious conditions, malignant pathology and vasculitic conditions is not appropriate since this is a known post-surgical complication.

30. Answer A

There are numerous techniques to reduce the inferior turbinates with long-standing debates on their efficacy. Surgery is generally considered once medical treatment has failed. A lateralisation/outfracture procedure should not be done in isolation. A randomised, prospective study concluded that submucosal resection of the cavernous tissue of the inferior turbinate with lateral displacement of the turbinate bone achieves a long-lasting improvement of the nasal passage with normalisation of the mucociliary transport time and without significant risk of post-operative bleeding.

Treatment of inferior turbinate hypertrophy: a randomised clinical trial. Passàli D et al, *Ann Otol Rhinol Laryngol.* 2003 Aug;112(8):683–8

31. Answer B

More lipophilic drugs like fluticasone have a longer elimination time. The systemic effects of intranasal corticosteroids have been widely studied and if used correctly, have not shown an increased incidence of hypothalamic-pituitary-adrenal (HPA) axis suppression, ocular symptoms or growth velocity adverse events. Fluticasone 17α esters such as fluticasone furoate and fluticasone propionate are stable, and their pharmacological activity is mediated by the entire molecule rather than either drug being a fluticasone prodrug.

32. Answer B

The effect of a single intravenous dose of corticosteroids (dexamethasone, 0.15–1.0 mg/kg) in paediatric tonsillectomy has been studied in a number of placebo-controlled trials. There is evidence that peri-operative dexamethasone reduces post-operative nausea and vomiting and early post-operative pain.

33. Answer A

Congenital midline craniofacial masses include nasal dermoids, gliomas and encephaloceles. Congenital nasal fistulas and dermoid cysts of the nose and frontal area are the most common of these rare congenital malformations. Fistulas may extend from the skin to the frontal bone or may extend through the skull base into the cranial cavity ending in an extradural cyst. They may also pass through the dura ending in a subarachnoid or intradural cyst. An MRI would be key to differentiate these and make a diagnosis. Management is surgical. If there is no intracranial extension there are several approaches that may be used including open rhinoplasty, transverse or vertical incision. In cases in which there is intracranial extension, a formal craniotomy will be required.

34. Answer C

During swallowing, the airway is protected by laryngeal elevation, closure of the true and false cords and by the cough reflex via sensory nerves located on the larynx, even prior to any aspiration event. The cuneiforms provide support to the vocal folds but are not directly involved in glottic closure.

35. Answer B

The anatomy of the paediatric airway differs from the adult.

- The paediatric tongue is larger relative to the size of the oral cavity.
- The paediatric larynx is more superior C1-C4 vs C4-C7 in adults.
- The paediatric epiglottis is larger and floppier. It is omega-shaped and angled more obliquely to the trachea.
- The smallest cross-sectional area in infants is at the subglottis whilst it is at the glottis (rima glottidis) in adults.

The postnasal space may be totally obstructed by adenoids in older children and hence the narrowest part of their airway. However, in neonates adenoids are not usually overly developed, meaning that generally the subglottis is the narrowest part of the airway.

36. Answer C

The Cotton-Myer grading scale is widely used for classifying the severity of subglottic stenosis and is as follows:

Grade I: up to 50% airway obstruction

Grade II: from 51% to 70% airway obstruction

Grade III: from 71% to 99% airway obstruction

Grade IV: no detectable lumen

It refers to the surface area of the stenosis. Staging is based on sizing the child's larynx with different endotracheal tubes and comparing this with reference tables of age-appropriate endotracheal tube sizes.

37. Answer E

Jehovah's Witnesses and the children for whom they are responsible may refuse consent to blood product administration due to their religious beliefs. This should be respected in an adult patient with capacity or those with an advanced directive. Children under 16 can give consent if they are deemed to be 'Gillick' competent—a child has sufficient competence if they are deemed to have the maturity and understanding to be capable of making decisions about their own health and medical treatment. It is judged on an individual basis. Refusal of treatment can be overridden in life-threatening emergencies, as is the case here. It could be considered that the child may be refusing because they are not in a good state of mind from the blood loss. A surgeon may be vulnerable to criminal prosecution if death of a minor may have been avoided with administration of blood.

A Specific Issue Order can be made under Section 8 of the Children Act 1989 to administer blood without removing all parental authority. If planning surgery and blood transfusion it is recommended that all efforts should be made to obtain a court order; however, due to the clinical urgency in this case, there is likely insufficient time to obtain this from a court.

The Jehovah's Witness Liaison Committee (JWLC) serves as a contact between patients who are Jehovah's Witnesses and healthcare providers. They provide support and guidance and advocate for patients whilst respecting their religious beliefs. They can be contacted by the patient or on behalf of the treating team. It would be recommended in this situation to speak with the JWLC who can assist in explaining the legal position to the family, but given the child's instability delaying treatment until they arrive would not be warranted.

38. Answer D

Hennebert's sign describes pressure-induced nystagmus and vertigo; a positive fistula test results in Hennebert's sign. Aquino's sign is the decrease in pulsation of paraganglioma with carotid artery compression. Hitselberger's sign describes numbness of the ear canal in response to CNVII compromise from vestibular schwannoma. Schwartze sign refers to the red hue behind the tympanic membrane, from hyperaemia of the promontory mucosa from increased vascularity, which represents the active phase of otosclerosis. The Tullio phenomenon is vertigo and nystagmus induced by loud sounds.

39. Answer E

The most common histological subtype of rhabdomyosarcoma is embryonal accounting for 75% of cases within the head and neck (either classical, botryoid or fusocellular). It is more common in infants and young children and is associated with the best prognosis. Alveolar rhabdomyosarcoma comprises 20% of cases, is more common in adolescence and has the worst prognosis. Pleomorphic rhabdomyosarcoma comprises 5% of cases and is more common in adults.

40. Answer B

Enlarged vestibular aqueduct (EVA) is associated with early-onset sensorineural hearing loss which is typically progressive (can be fluctuating) with variable vestibular symptoms. Hearing loss is known to worsen after head trauma. EVA can be associated with other cochleovestibular abnormalities and may be found in isolation or as part of a syndrome. It is diagnosed on CT or MRI with a vestibular aqueduct diameter >1.5 mm at the midpoint between the common crus and operculum. It is associated with Mondini dysplasia, Pendred syndrome and branchio-oto-renal syndrome. Genes associated with non-syndromic EVA include *SLC26A4* and *FOXI1*. Treatment is conservative with advice to avoid head trauma (avoid contact sports/judicious use of helmet) and hearing rehabilitation.

41. Answer C

Usher's syndrome results in sensorineural hearing loss and progressive loss of vision due to retinitis pigmentosa. There are different clinical types: I – congenital bilateral profound hearing loss and absent vestibular function, II – moderate hearing loss and normal vestibular function, III – progressive hearing loss and variable vestibular dysfunction. Pendred's syndrome is autosomal recessive in inheritance. Jervell and Lange-Nielsen syndrome results from mutations affecting a potassium channel gene. Apert syndrome, an acrocephalosyndactyly, is associated with the *FGFR2* gene and is not X-linked. Waardenburg syndrome is associated with sensorineural hearing loss.

42. Answer E

Alport syndrome is caused by an X-lined mutation in type IV collagen gene (*COL45*). Dysfunctional basement membrane collagen in the inner ear, eye and kidney result in progressive hearing loss, kidney disease (glomerulonephritis) and eye disease (lenticonus, keratoconus, cataracts and corneal erosion). Since it is an X-linked recessive disorder, females are typically carriers of the mutation, and the severity of their symptoms can vary.

43. Answer C

Bilateral nasal polyposis in a young child is concerning for cystic fibrosis (CF). CF is an autosomal recessive condition caused by mutations in the cystic fibrosis transmembrane conductance regulator gene (CFTR). To date over 700 mutations have been identified in the gene with delta F508 accounting for 70% of cases. These mutations result in the formation of thick sticky secretions impairing mucous clearance culminating in bacterial colonisation. Detection of elevated sweat chloride values (greater than 60 mmol/L) by quantitative pilocarpine iontophoresis test (sweat test) is the gold standard diagnostic test. Management of nasal polyps is with corticosteroids, regular sinus irrigations and endoscopic sinus surgery. A CT scan should be performed for pre-operative planning because it helps localise and define the extent of disease, but the priority in this case is to rule out or make a diagnosis of cystic fibrosis.

44. Answer A

The steeple sign is a radiologic sign referring to the tapering of the upper trachea, representing subglottic narrowing/oedema on an AP view of a chest radiograph which resembles a church steeple. It is suggestive of croup. Double ring or halo sign refers to the two concentric circles corresponding to the two metallic discs that make up button batteries and is therefore indicative of button battery ingestion. Holman-Miller sign refers to the anterior bowing of the posterior wall of the maxillary sinus as seen on a lateral skull radiograph or cross-sectional imaging. It is seen in juvenile nasopharyngeal angiofibroma. Thumbprint sign is seen on lateral soft-tissue radiograph of the neck and is a manifestation of an oedematous and enlarged epiglottis suggestive of epiglottitis.

45. Answer D

Diagnosis of atypical mycobacterial lymphadenitis is usually clinical. It may be suspected followed failed antibiotic therapy aimed at Staphylococcus and Streptococcus or persistence with conservative treatment for presumed viral aetiology. Eventually, spontaneous drainage or fistulae occur. Culture and sensitivity may be diagnostic (requires 2–4 weeks). PCR is more sensitive. Tuberculin skin testing is a nonspecific method to confirm infection; however, it may be weak or negative. Incision and drainage should be avoided due to high probability of recurrence and fistula formation. Full surgical excision is superior to medical therapy but may be complicated by facial nerve damage.

46. Answer C

Congenital tracheoesophageal fistula is a result of failure of recannulation of the oesophagus or developmental failure of the tracheoesophageal septum. There are various types: oesophageal atresia with distal tracheoesophageal fistula is the most common (85%, and hence the most likely in this scenario) followed by isolated oesophageal atresia without tracheoesophageal fistula (~ 10%). Clinical features include cyanosis and gagging, vomiting, abdominal distension, drooling, cough, recurrent aspiration pneumonia and feeding difficulties. The diagnosis is suggested when an NGT is passed and meets obstruction at 9–13 cm. Radiographs may demonstrate a gas-filled GI tract and often right upper lobe pneumonia (aspiration). Contrast swallow is diagnostic.

47. Answer B

Laryngo-tracheo-oesophageal defects including laryngeal clefts are a result of failure of the tracheoesophageal septum to develop. Symptoms depend on the severity of the cleft and include respiratory distress at birth, stridor, aspiration, recurrent pneumonia and dysphagia. Congenital syndromes associated with laryngeal clefts include Opitz G/BBB, Pallister-Hall, CHARGE, VATER/VACTERL. Other associated congenital abnormalities include tracheomalacia, tracheoesophageal fistula and congenital cardiac defects. The gold standard for diagnosis is suspension microlaryngoscopy and bronchoscopy. A small laryngeal cleft may be missed on barium swallow, CXR or video-fluroscopy. Similarly, if MLB is performed without palpation, a laryngeal cleft may be missed.

48. Answer B

Furstenberg's sign is a clinical finding seen in masses of the head, such as a meningocele, that communicate with the intracranial compartment. Due to the intracranial communication, there is an increase in size of the mass with increases in intracranial pressure such as occurs with compression of the internal jugular vein or Valsalva. Meningoceles change in size with straining and crying, are compressible and transilluminate. Gliomas and dermoids do not change in size with straining and crying, are noncompressible and do not transilluminate. These lesions are Furstenberg negative.

49. Answer D

Laryngomalacia is the most common cause of congenital stridor. Stridor is exacerbated with crying and feeding or when supine. It is usually self-limiting and resolves by 18–24 months. Indications for surgical intervention include poor weight gain, failure to thrive and apnoeic spells. Supraglottoplasty is the mainstay of surgical treatment. Aryepiglottoplasty is a variant of supraglottoplasty and involves the division of the aryepiglottic folds close the base of the epiglottis, allowing the epiglottis to unfurl and reduce the airway obstruction.

50. Answer A

Neck stiffness raises suspicion of a retropharyngeal abscess. It usually occurs in children under the age of 5. It is often preceded by an upper respiratory tract infection, involving the retropharyngeal lymph nodes (of Rouvière) which drain the nasopharynx, adenoids, sinuses and middle ear, leading to suppurative cervical lymphadenitis and a retropharyngeal abscess. Neck stiffness is not typical for epiglottitis and patients may adopt a 'sniffing' (neck extension) posture. Trismus is an important clinical indicator of peritonsillar abscess due to the associated inflammation of the pterygoid muscles.

51. Answer C

Lemierre syndrome is characterised by thrombophlebitis of the internal jugular vein(s) and disseminated septic emboli following oropharyngeal infection. It usually affects previously healthy adolescents and young adults. It is typically caused by *Fusobacterium necrophorum*, either as a primary infection or as a fusobacterial super-infection. The 'cord sign' is an induration of the internal jugular vein at the angle of the mandible. Treatment is with broad spectrum antibiotics and may require admission to ITU for organ support. The role of anti-coagulation in these patients is controversial but may be warranted with large clot burden or spread to the intracranial dural sinuses.

52. Answer A

Bilateral choanal atresia presents in newborns with cyclical cyanosis/apnoea which resolves with crying since neonates are obligate nasal breathers. It should be treated as a medical emergency with the priority to secure the airway with an oropharyngeal airway or McGovern nipple. If there is no improvement there should be a low threshold for orotracheal intubation. Clinical evaluation includes introducing a suction catheter through each nostril, flexible nasendoscopy and using a laryngeal mirror under the nostril to check for misting. CT scan confirms diagnosis and extent of atresia. Other investigations include looking for associated anomalies (e.g. CHARGE syndrome). Management is endoscopic or transpalatal surgical repair +/- stents.

53. Answer D

CHARGE syndrome is the most common concurrent syndrome associated with cho-anal atresia. The acronym stands for **C**oloboma, **H**eart disease, **A**tresia (choanal), **R**etardation (CNS), **G**enital hypoplasia and **E**ar anomalies (outer, middle and inner). Inner ear anomalies including the Mondini malformation (incomplete partition type II and large vestibular aqueduct) and semicircular canal agenesis are common and associated with sensorineural hearing loss and vestibular dysfunction. Mondini malformation is also associated with Pendred, Klippel-Feil, DiGeorge and Windervanck syndromes.

54. Answer C

The rate of acute otitis media complicated with facial nerve palsy has decreased given the widespread use of antibiotics. Aggressive IV antimicrobial therapy with urgent myringotomy, with or without grommet placement, to allow the suppurative process to drain is required for treatment. Culture of the middle ear fluid should be performed. If there are signs of abscess or coalescent mastoiditis, mastoidectomy should be performed. In cases in which there is concern for intracranial complications, or corti-cal mastoidectomy is planned, then CT imaging is indicated. In this case a CT scan is warranted because the child is irritable, and it is difficult to assess neurology in young children. Additionally, since the child is going to theatre for a grommet, then other pathology such as an intracranial collection should be dealt with at this time. Facial nerve decompression is not warranted initially since most cases of infection-related facial palsy will improve with treatment of the infection.

55. Answer C

The diagnosis of peritonsillar abscess is usually clinical. Predominant physical examina-tion findings include trismus, deviation of the uvula to the contralateral side, ipsilateral bulge of the soft palate and anterior pillar and an enlarged medially displaced tonsil.

CT is the imaging modality of choice to confirm the diagnosis and is indicated in select cases including uncooperative children, severe trismus preventing clinical examination, diagnostic uncertainty, concern of development of a complication and persistence despite optimal treatment.

56. Answer E

A congenital piriform sinus fistula from a third branchial arch origin penetrates the cricothyroid muscle and terminates in the thyroid gland. Infection manifests as recurrent acute thyroid or neck abscess. After incision and drainage of the abscess, definitive treatment requires formal excision of the fistulous tract which may include hemithyroidectomy. It should be noted that fourth arch anomalies can present similarly.

57. Answer D

In this case there is a highly suggestive history of foreign body aspiration. The majority of aspirated foreign bodies in children are radiolucent food items. Even in the absence of physical signs the history and witnessed coughing is persuasive enough to warrant rigid bronchoscopy under general anaesthetic.

58. Answer E

In children with bronchial foreign bodies, especially if there is evidence of respiratory distress or potential airway compromise, rigid bronchoscopy is the preferred intervention for foreign body retrieval. Rigid bronchoscopy allows for direct visualisation and the safe removal of the foreign body under direct vision whilst also allowing the airway to be secured (which is not directly possible with flexible bronchoscopy). The timing of the procedure is more debateable. The child is stable in a monitored environment and given the practical concerns of organising a paediatric theatre with suitably trained staff overnight, it is reasonable and safe to delay removal until the next day.

Removal of inhaled foreign bodies—middle of the night or the next morning?

Mani N et al, *Int J Pediatr Otorhinolaryngol* 2009 Aug;73(8):1085–9

59. Answer C

Subglottic haemangiomas are effectively treated by propranolol, with success rates >85%. Non-responders are rare but been reported. Children commencing propranolol therapy require close monitoring since side effects include hypotension, bradycardia, hypoglycaemia, peripheral vasoconstriction, fatigue and bronchospasm. Prior to commencing propranolol therapy, it is recommended that an electrocardiogram is performed. Echocardiogram may be requested based on the history but is generally not required since structural heart disease has not been associated with isolated subglottic haemangioma.

60. Answer D

In a child with a retropharyngeal abscess that is under 2 cm without stridor/stertor or respiratory distress that has not received a trial of IV antibiotics (24–48 hours), a recommendation for intubation by paediatric anaesthesia would not be appropriate. If this is not the case and surgical drainage is considered, then this can either be via the oral or transcervical approach depending on the location of the abscess. In this case given that the oral examination was normal the transcervical case may be warranted. The transcervical approach also has the advantage of providing gravity-dependent drainage of the abscess cavity.

61. Answer A

Children have a 'cone'-shaped airway with the subglottis at the apex, making it the narrowest portion of the airway.

62. Answer E

Poiseuille's law (the Hagen–Poiseuille equation) states that airway resistance is inversely proportional to the fourth power of its radius. Therefore, a 50% reduction in the radius of the airway results in a 16-fold increase in resistance to airflow.

63. Answer D

Paediatric subglottic stenosis can be congenital or acquired; however, most subglottic stenosis is due to intubation injury related to traumatic or prolonged intubations.

64. Answer B

When assessing stridor, one is required to note the onset and duration with respect to the respiratory cycle (inspiratory vs expiratory vs biphasic). Biphasic stridor is classic of glottic/subglottic pathology. Supraglottic pathology classically has inspiratory stridor, and intrathoracic pathology usually has expiratory stridor.

65. Answer A

The left recurrent laryngeal nerve has a more descending/extensive course and is therefore more prone to injury during cardiothoracic surgery. Children therefore usually present with hoarseness and on flexible laryngoscopy, usually have left vocal cord palsy.

66. Answer E

When sizing the airway, an uncuffed endotracheal tube that is expected to pass without resistance or expansion is placed and connected to the anaesthesia circuit. The pressure is brought up gradually within the airway while simultaneously observing for a leak around the endotracheal tube. If the endotracheal tube has a free leak or leaks at a low pressure (<5–10 cmH$_2$0), the next size (larger) endotracheal tube can be placed and assessed. A correctly sized tube will have a leak at 20 cmH$_2$0. Pressures are generally not brought above 25 cmH$_2$0 during this assessment.

67. Answer C

Children who are likely to respond well to this technique usually have thin or web-like and soft stenoses consisting of immature scar tissue. Dilation is less likely to yield positive outcomes in longer stenoses, those with thick mature scar tissue and in patients with additional airway lesions.

68. Answer E

During MLB patients are required to be breathing spontaneously to allow an assessment of the airway without need for intubation and ventilation. Therefore, muscle paralysis is not given. Oxygen can be supplemented via an endotracheal tube held in the pharynx.

69. Answer A

One of the goals of laryngotracheal reconstruction (LTR) is to avoid a tracheostomy or to allow decannulation. If the patient does not have a tracheostomy in situ then they can have a single stage LTR. Patients with a tracheostomy can have a single or double staged LTR. If results of a sleep evaluation indicate pulmonary or neurological compromise that precludes decannulation, this pathology may need to be addressed prior to laryngeal reconstruction.

70. Answer A

Laryngeal keels were developed and used to prevent problematic anterior commissure re-stenosis/webs. Keel placement can be endoscopic or open requiring laryngofissure.

71. Answer C

Congenital stenosis results from a failure or incomplete recanalisation of the laryngotracheal tube during the third month of gestation and may lead to a spectrum of laryngeal anomalies such as laryngeal atresia, webs and subglottic stenosis. In congenital subglottic stenosis, symptoms generally appear shortly after birth (biphasic stridor, dyspnoea, sternal recessions).

72. Answer B

Awake flexible laryngoscopy has the main advantage of assessing dynamic laryngeal movement that allows assessment of the supraglottis (e.g. for laryngomalacia) and for vocal fold movement. However, it is generally not possible to go through the vocal folds in an awake child since this may lead to life-threatening laryngospasm, and therefore views of the subglottis are limited.

73. Answer C

Laryngotracheal reconstruction can fail and may ultimately require a tracheostomy. Myer-Cotton grade 3 and anterior and posterior subglottic stenosis, providing the patient is a suitable candidate, can be managed with laryngotracheal reconstruction.

74. Answer E

Tragal cartilage is too limited and weak to be considered as a graft for airway reconstruction. The primary source of cartilage used for this purpose is costal cartilage which is considered to have the strongest properties. This is followed in frequency by thyroid alar cartilage, and auricular cartilage (rare). Tragal cartilage should not be used.

75. Answer D

Laryngotracheal reconstruction can be performed at a single stage, using the endotracheal tube as a temporary stent after surgery, or in multiple stages, with a tracheostomy inserted (if not already in place) to safeguard the airway post-operatively.

76. Answer C

Passavant's ridge is formed by the superior pharyngeal constrictor muscle fibres creating an anterior displacement of the posterior pharyngeal wall. It is an important structure in maintaining velopharyngeal competence. In this case the adenoidectomy is indicated because of obstructive sleep apnoea; however, it should aim to maintain Passavant's ridge and its surrounding adenoidal tissue. The adenoidal tissue obstructing the choanae superiorly can be safely taken down. Performing an adenoidectomy without maintaining Passavant's ridge will increase the risk of post-adenoidectomy velopharyngeal insufficiency.

77. Answer C

Only children with a cleft with a palatal component will be more prone to developing ETD due to the abnormal insertions of the levator veli palatini and tensor veli palatini.

Timing of the placement of ventilation tubes is controversial but usually these are performed at the time of cleft palate repair.

78. Answer A

The Haberman design allows the feeding to be activated by pressure (from tongue, gum) rather than sucking which is impaired in this population.

79. Answer C

Recurrent respiratory papillomatosis is typified by recurrent exophytic papilloma of the epithelial mucosa of the respiratory tract caused by infection with human papillomavirus types 6 and 11. Treatment is primarily surgical including microdebrider, cold steel instruments and laser excision. Adjuvant therapies are recommended in children undergoing frequent surgical procedures (3–4 procedures a year is often used a guide). There is no agreed first-line medication in the UK, but most centres will now prefer Avastin (Bevacizumab) over Cidofovir.

80. Answer D

In the absence of red flag symptoms or signs (e.g. stridor, dyspnoea, cyanosis) that would necessitate MLB, referral for speech therapy is appropriate. Speech therapy can help assess and address any functional issues related to voice production, especially in a child who is actively engaged in singing. If there is no improvement with speech therapy or if symptoms persist or worsen, further investigations may be considered.

81. Answer C

The most likely cause of voice change in children with long term tracheostomy is suprastomal granulation. This is the formation of granulation tissue above the tracheostomy stoma. This granulation tissue can impact the airflow through the upper airway and affect vocal quality.

82. Answer E

Prominent ears typically become noticeable in early childhood and may be a source of child and parental anxiety. Corrective surgery should consider factors such as auricular growth, cartilage flexibility and the age of the child. Typically, otoplasty surgery is not considered until after school age (5 years). Ear splinting is typically only effective in children under 18 months of age. It is appropriate to see the child again after he has begun school to both allow time for normal ear development and to make a fuller assessment of the psychological impacts of prominauris.

83. Answer D

This action ensures that suspicions are communicated to a team specialised in child health and potentially child protection, who can then take further steps, including a thorough examination for other injuries, further investigations and involving social services if necessary. It's imperative to follow local and centre guidelines on reporting and managing suspected cases of non-accidental injury to ensure the child's safety and well-being.

84. Answer A

The clinical scenario is suggestive of an atypical mycobacterial infection. These non-tuberculous mycobacteria are commonly found in the environment, including in soil and water, and can sometimes cause infections in children under 5 and the immunocompromised. Typically, these present as an enlarging neck mass with violaceous discolouration of the overlying skin that does not respond to antibiotics. The most definitive treatment is complete surgical excision; however, because of the risks to underlying neurovascular structure, a prolonged course of antibiotics is often trialled, but this may take many months to take effect. The typical histopathology finding is caseating granulomas with central necrosis and multinucleated giant cells. Non-caseating granulomas are formed in inflammatory conditions such as sarcoidosis, Crohn's disease and foreign body reactions. Orphan Annie nuclei, a term coined by Dr. Nancy E. Warner (professor of pathology at the University of Southern California, USA) describes characteristically empty nuclei seen in malignant conditions including papillary thyroid cancer and autoimmune thyroiditis.

85. Answer A

Sensorineural hearing loss, visual deterioration (retinitis pigmentosa) and vestibular abnormalities in the first decade of life are typical of Usher syndrome (type 1). The condition is caused by mutations in one of several genes: *CDH23*, *MYO7A*, *PCDH15*, *USH1C* and *USH1G* and display autosomal recessive inheritance. Usher type 2 patients have a less significant hearing loss and lose vision in the second decade. Balance abnormalities are not found in Usher type 2. The condition results from mutations in *USH2A*, *GRP98* or *DFNB31*. Usher syndrome type 3 is like type 1, but the phenotype is milder and results from mutation in *CLRN1*.

86. Answer B

Although currently stable the inspiratory stridor is evidence of an airway injury which has the potential to evolve. Observation in the ED allows for further assessment and monitoring of the patient's respiratory status. Securing of the airway would be considered if there is a deterioration in the patient's respiratory status. However, the initial approach is to closely observe the patient and provide supportive care. Admission to paediatric ITU may be warranted if respiratory support is required.

87. Answer C

Everyone over 16 is presumed to be able to provide consent unless they lack capacity. Children under 16 may be able to consent for their own treatment if they are deemed able to understand the proposed treatment (Gillick competence). Children under 16 years cannot refuse treatment that has been agreed by someone with parental responsibility or the court and is in their best interest. Generally parental responsibility lies with the child's birth parents. People with parental responsibility include the birth mother, the birth father if married to the mother at the time of birth or the child's father (for those born after 1 Dec 2003) if his name is on the birth certificate. Additionally, those named on the birth certificate, legal guardians and the local authority if appointed by the court can also consent. In this case, the biological father is present and they were married at the time of the child's birth, so he is able to consent to the procedure.

88. Answer D

At age 8–10 years, there are multiple factors that facilitate surgery: the other (normal) pinna has grown enough and reaches adult size, allowing the reconstruction to achieve the best and most stable symmetry. There is also enough rib cartilage available that needs to be thick and robust enough. Lastly, waiting until this age allows the child's ability to be a part of the decision and hence be an active participant.

89. Answer D

An absent cochlear nerve is an absolute contraindication for cochlear implantation; the rest, apart from additional surgical considerations, are not absolute contraindications.

90. Answer D

Incidence of congenital tracheal stenosis (CTS) is estimated to be 1 in 64,500 births, and accounts for only 0.1% to 0.3% of all types of laryngotracheal stenosis. The most common cause of CTS is complete tracheal rings with a greater incidence in trisomy 21 or VACTERL.

91. Answer E

Obstructive sleep apnoea in children with trisomy 21 is multifactorial and secondary to multiple factors: midface and mandibular hypoplasia, narrow nasopharynx, muscle hypotonia, macroglossia/glossoptosis, lingual tonsillar hypertrophy, laryngomalacia, usual adenotonsillar hypertrophy and a propensity for obesity.

92. Answer D

Approximately 63% of patients with trisomy 21 who have persistent OSA following adenotonsillectomy have glossoptosis. Sites to look out for in refractory OSA are base-of-tongue obstruction, pharyngeal collapse, crowding associated with obesity and lingual tonsil hypertrophy.

93. Answer A

During each breath, the system delivers a signal to the hypoglossal nerve which activates upper airway muscles, predominantly the genioglossus muscle, thereby opening the airway to prevent obstructive events.

94. Answer C

ABEPs are neurophysiological responses that reflect the electrical activity generated in the auditory nerve and brainstem in response to auditory stimuli. The most clinically informative metrics from an ABR are the wave latencies, amplitudes and interwave intervals between waves I to III, III to V, and I to V. Latencies are correlated with age, reflecting maturation of the auditory axis, and intensity of stimulation. Latencies are generally longer in neonates and shorten with age. Components II, IV and VI of ABEPs are typically not well defined before the age of 32–36 weeks in preterm infants. Wave V latency and interpeak latencies are generally longer in premature infants reflecting the immaturity of the auditory axis.

95. Answer B

A compensatory tachycardia in response to blood volume loss is an attempt to maintain cardiac output. A 15% loss of blood volume is sufficient to trigger this response in a child (Class II shock). Class I <15% blood volume loss, Class III 30–40%, Class IV >40%.

In children blood volume is approximately 75 ml/kg, so for a 20 kg child the blood volume would be 1500 ml. A 15% blood volume loss would be approximately 225 ml.

96. **Answer C**

    Laryngeal cleft is a rare congenital abnormality characterised by abnormal commu-
    nication between the respiratory system at the level of the larynx and trachea and
    oesophagus. It is due to failure of the tracheoesophageal septum to form. Various
    classifications have been proposed with the Benjamin Inglis classification the most
    recognised. There are 4 types – Type I: supraglottic interarytenoid defect; Type II: par-
    tial cricoid involvement with extension below the level of the true vocal cords; Type III:
    complete cricoid cleft into the cervical trachea; Type IV: cleft extending beyond the
    thoracic inlet to involve the thoracic trachea.

97. **Answer C**

    Post-grommet infection is one of the most common complications of grommet inser-
    tion. Ciprofloxacin drops are the best treatment option since systemic antibiotics will
    not eradicate the biofilm on the grommet. Treatment failure will occasionally neces-
    sitate removal and/or changing of the grommet.

98. **Answer E**

    Usher syndrome is the most common cause of autosomal recessive hearing loss. It
    results in sensorineural hearing loss and progressive loss of vision due to retinitis pig-
    mentosa. There are 3 different clinical types – I: congenital bilateral profound hearing
    loss and absent vestibular function; II: moderate hearing loss and normal vestibular
    function; III: progressive hearing loss and variable vestibular dysfunction. Jervell and
    Lange-Nielsen syndrome results from mutations affecting a potassium channel gene.

99. **Answer A**

    The diagnosis is consistent with juvenile-onset recurrent respiratory papillomatosis. CT
    chest should be considered to evaluate pulmonary involvement particularly in cases
    of distal tracheal disease. Whilst spread of disease to the distal tracheobronchial tree
    is rare it carries a poor prognosis.

100. **Answer D**

    The presence of skin telangiectasia suggests a vascular component to the lesion mak-
    ing a first branchial arch anomaly less likely. Parotid gland haemangiomas constitute
    50% of paediatric parotid gland tumours. They may occur as part of segmental V3
    haemangioma or be an isolated focal haemangioma. They are congenital and
    undergo a rapid proliferative growth phase followed by involution. They are treated
    with oral propranolol. Pleomorphic adenoma is unlikely in this age group and as
    regards paediatric presentation it typically occurs in adolescents. It presents as a
    slow-growing, painless mass without skin changes. Acute or chronic inflammatory/
    infectious diseases are the predominant cause of parotid swelling in children; how-
    ever, the clinical history does not fit with acute parotitis. Mucoepidermoid carcinoma
    represents 50% of all malignant parotid tumours and generally occurs between 5 and
    15 years, so is unlikely in this clinical scenario.

CHAPTER 4: RHINOLOGY AND FACIAL PLASTIC SURGERY

1. You are referred a 53-year-old female with clear right-sided nasal drip and intermittent headaches by her general practitioner (GP). She has no trauma history, has never had sinonasal surgery and has no allergy history. She has tried nasal sprays and drops but they have not helped. She feels that the drip tastes salty. The beta-trace-protein testing of the fluid is positive, which is highly suggestive of a CSF leak. She has changes in her vision and thus prior to repairing the defect, you refer her to the neuro-ophthalmologist. What is the most likely visual field defect on examination?
   A Central scotoma
   B Bitemporal hemianopia
   C Macular sparing defect
   D Enlarged blind spot
   E Superior quadrantinopia

2. You review a 55-year-old male in clinic who has significant nasal blockage, catarrh, congestion and hyposmia. Nasendoscopy did not demonstrate the presence of polyps, but a CT scan reveals pan-sinus opacification with inflammatory changes. He has not responded well to intranasal rinsing and topical steroids for three months but is not keen on surgery. You decide to prescribe a three-month trial of antibiotics according to the EPOS 2020 (European Position Paper on Rhinosinusitis and Nasal Polyps 2020) guidelines and therefore organise an ECG prior to commencing therapy.

What ECG changes can be precipitated by the most appropriate prescribed antibiotic?
   A Prolonged PR interval
   B Prolonged QT interval
   C QRS narrowing
   D QRS widening
   E T-wave abnormalities

3. You review a 37-year-old male who has significant nasal congestion and a nasal deformity following trauma to the nose several years ago. He has a C-shaped external deformity, with a significant septal deviation bilaterally, with reduced airflow. There is alar collapse on inspiration which is aided with a Cottle manoeuvre. He does not have any allergies on skin prick allergy testing and denies any history of sinusitis. He has not had any benefit with nasal douching or intranasal steroids. What surgical procedure is the most appropriate for this patient?
   A Septoplasty and turbinoplasty
   B Endonasal septorhinoplasty
   C External septorhinoplasty with osteotomies
   D External septorhinoplasty with spreader grafts
   E External septorhinoplasty with spreader grafts and alar batten graft

4. A 48-year-old female comes to see you with a change in the shape of her nose after having a cosmetic rhinoplasty abroad three years ago. Her nasal function is largely unchanged,

DOI: 10.1201/9781003455059-4

although she has some worsening of her nasal blockage compared to immediately after the procedure. Her external profile is unremarkable, and within the midline, with minimal impairment of nasal flow. On reviewing the operation notes she brings to clinic, you note the previous surgeon has documented that they performed an external septorhinoplasty with osteotomies and a de-hump. The upper lateral cartilages were divided, but there is no clear documentation of re-attachment to the nasal septum. What is the most likely deformity she is presenting with to your clinic?

A Pollybeak deformity
B Saddle nose deformity
C Inverted V deformity
D Ptotic tip deformity
E Pseudo-hump deformity

5. A 39-year-old female has been referred to your rhinology clinic with nasal obstruction, crusting, intermittent epistaxis and irritation. She has not noticed any change to the external appearance of her nose and denies previous surgery. On examination you note significant nasal crusting with an anterior septal perforation and an eschar. What is the most common cause of septal perforation in the UK?

A Septal surgery
B Cocaine misuse
C Digital/local trauma
D Granulomatous disease
E Malignancy

6. A 62-year-old South Asian female is referred to you from your local orbital MDT because of an infero-medial orbital lesion extending into the pterygopalatine fossae. She presented to ophthalmology with eye pain and pressure, reduced visual acuity and some mild proptosis. The lesion requires tissue biopsy and has been referred for an endoscopic endonasal approach.

Which of the following nerves is most at risk of injury during this procedure?

A Optic nerve
B Infraorbital nerve
C Ophthalmic nerve
D Maxillary nerve
E Mandibular nerve

7. A 5-year-old boy presents to the emergency department with a new-onset forehead swelling and fever on a background of a recent coryzal illness over the past two weeks. He is diagnosed with a Pott's puffy tumour and subsequently has an admission to hospital for intravenous antibiotics, analgesia, fluids and imaging prior to surgery later that day. Microbiology swabs are taken at the time of operation and tissue samples are also sent for analysis. What is the most likely organism to be grown from the specimens?

A *Staphylococcus aureus*
B *Moraxella catarrhalis*
C *Streptococcus pneumoniae*
D *Haemophilus influenzae*
E Fusobacterium

8. A 17-year-old male is referred to your clinic with a longstanding nasal congestion, particularly in the spring, which has not responded to treatment in the community. He has a strong family history of atopy and allergies. He also suffers from asthma, which is reasonably well controlled at present. His skin prick allergy test is positive for house dust mites, grasses and pollen. He has an elevated serum IgE level. Exam shows inferior turbinate hypertrophy and a midline septum. The patient expresses relief in his symptoms after decongestion. When should the patient be offered surgery to reduce the size of his turbinates?

A He is a candidate right now and surgery is best option for him to manage his nasal obstruction
B After failing a trial of topical corticosteroids and topical antihistamines

C After a failed trial of oral antihistamines

D After received subcutaneous immunotherapy for 5 years with no improvement

E When medical therapy does not reduce his IgE levels to the normal range

9. **A 58-year-old driving instructor is referred to you because of worsening snoring with suspected obstructive sleep apnoea (OSA). He has a high body mass index (BMI) and a large neck circumference (collar size 17.5). Examination reveals mild rhinitis with a mildly deviated septum with no significant obstruction. He has not benefitted from topical steroid therapy and feels his symptoms are worsening and affecting his ability to work. Which of the following findings is most likely to be associated with severe OSA?**
   A Large neck circumference
   B High BMI
   C Daytime activity being affected
   D Hypertension
   E Narcolepsy

10. **You are referred a 53-year-old female with right-sided nasal drip by her GP. She denies any history of trauma, sinus surgery or allergy. She has trialled topical steroid therapy without relief. Beta-2-transferrin/tau protein analysis is positive, which is suggestive of a CSF leak. Which condition can lead to a false positive beta-2-transferrin test of nasal secretions?**
    A Granulomatosis with polyangiitis
    B Sarcoidosis
    C Tuberculosis
    D Chronic alcoholism
    E Parkinson's disease

11. **A 32-year-old man presents to your clinic complaining of chronic nasal obstruction. On examination, you note a deviated septum and a notably narrow piriform aperture. He has a history**

of nasal trauma. Which surgical option would be most beneficial if you were to proceed with a septorhinoplasty?
   A Alar batten grafts
   B Caudal septal extension graft
   C Spreader grafts
   D Columellar strut
   E Butterfly graft

12. **You are in otology clinic and are reviewing a 65-year-old female who last year underwent a rhytidectomy. She tells you that over the last year she has developed considerable shooting pains in her left ear and the pain is significantly exacerbated in the cold. Which nerve has most likely been injured as a result of the surgery?**
    A Great auricular nerve injury
    B Marginal mandibular nerve injury
    C Greater occipital nerve
    D Auriculotemporal nerve
    E Lesser occipital nerve

13. **A 31-year-old male who has recently immigrated from Indonesia attends the emergency department due to worsening nasal pain, crusting, congestion, bleeding and facial fullness. He has a long history of nasal obstruction and rhinorrhoea, but this has significantly worsened over the past 6 weeks. On examination he has scarring, crusting, adhesions and thick purulent mucus in both nasal cavities. You suspect he has rhinoscleroma and start him on antibiotics, nasal rinsing, antibiotic topical ointments and topical steroids. Which imaging modality is best to assess the extent of the disease?**
    A CT sinuses without contrast
    B CT sinuses with contrast
    C T1 MRI with contrast
    D T1 MRI without contrast
    E T2 MRI without contrast

14. **A 47-year-old patient on chemotherapy for acute lymphoblastic leukaemia (ALL) is referred with left eye swelling,**

worsening facial pain and head-ache. The on-call registrar assesses the patient and is concerned about orbital cellulitis. The patient can open their eye and initial examination of the vision is normal. Treatment with intrave-nous antibiotics and nasal rinsing with topical steroids is commenced. Two days later you are asked to review the patient because they have worsening symptoms and further increased serum infection markers. They have a worsen-ing headache and now both eyes seem to be affected. Which of the following is most likely to indicate evidence of cavernous sinus thrombosis?

A Swinging pyrexia
B Reduced Glasgow coma score (GCS)
C Proptosis of the eye(s)
D Facial nerve palsy
E Reduction in sensation in the trigemi-nal nerve distribution

15. You are reviewing a 27-year-old female with chronic rhinosinusitis with nasal polyposis (CRSwP). Despite nasal rins-ing and topical steroids, she remains congested. Flexible nasal endoscopy demonstrates grade 4 polyps bilater-ally. You decide to prescribe her a week of oral prednisolone whilst await-ing surgery. Which is the most common adverse effect of oral steroids that you should warn her about?

A Weight gain
B Thinning of the skin or skin pigmenta-tion changes
C Insomnia or nightmares
D Peptic ulcer disease
E Alopecia

16. A 72-year-old female with refractory hereditary haemorrhagic telangiecta-sia (HHT) is seeking further intervention for her recurrent epistaxis. She has had multiple laser procedures in the past and failed bilateral septodermoplasty, and is three months post nasal closure. She has ongoing intermittent bleeding into the oropharynx. She has required several admissions to hospital includ-ing blood transfusions. Your colleague suggests she might be a candidate for bevacizumab. What is the mechanism of action of this medication?

A Up regulation of vascular endothelial growth factor
B Down regulation of vascular endothe-lial growth factor
C TGF-ß1 signalling pathway enhance-ment of angiogenesis
D TGF-ß1 signalling pathway enhance-ment of vasospasm
E Pro-angiogenic cytokine in angiogenesis

17. You review a 32-year-old patient with known CRSwP who has significant sinus symptoms of mucus drip, hyposmia, congestion and facial pain. A CT scan reveals significant sinus disease and there has been limited benefit from topical nasal steroid therapy with nasal rinsing. You discuss surgery with the patient and are explaining the sinus drainage pathways to the medical student who is with you in clinic. Which of the following sinuses drains into the sphenoethmoidal recess?

A Anterior ethmoid
B Posterior ethmoid
C Frontal
D Maxillary
E All of the above

18. Which of the following is not a branch of the sphenopalatine artery?

A Inferior turbinate branch
B Posterior septal branch
C Palatovaginal artery
D Middle turbinate branch
E Posterolateral branch

19. A 70-year-old retired furniture factory worker is referred to your clinic with nasal congestion, blood-stained dis-charge and irritation. He has left aural fullness and otalgia with some muffling

of his hearing. You note he has a firm left-sided neck mass and flexible nasendoscopy reveals a left nasal cavity mass. What is the most likely diagnosis?
A Antrochoanal polyp
B Inverted papilloma
C Adenocarcinoma
D Adenoid cystic carcinoma
E Squamous cell carcinoma

20. You are about to perform endoscopic sinus surgery in a 47-year-old female with CRSwNP. In the theatre brief you ask the anaesthetist to spray some co-phenylcaine spray pre-operatively to aid decongestion. How much lignocaine is in a standard vial of co-phenylcaine spray?
A 50 mg
B 75 mg
C 100 mg
D 125 mg
E 150 mg

21. A 19-year-old Afro-Caribbean female presents with keloid scarring at the site of a cosmetic pinna piercing. In the management of keloid scarring on the pinna, which of the following treatment modalities is considered a first-line option for reducing keloid size and symptoms?
A Excision with primary closure
B Intralesional corticosteroid injections
C Laser therapy
D Silicone gel sheets
E Radiation therapy

22. An elderly man presents with a scaly lesion on the forehead that is clinically a squamous cell carcinoma (SCC). What is the appropriate excision margin for a squamous cell carcinoma located on the face?
A 1–2 mm
B 4–6 mm
C 10–12 mm
D 20–22 mm
E 30–32 mm

23. A 14-year-old boy is referred urgently to your clinic with left-sided facial pain, nasal congestion and a post-nasal drip. He also has a left-sided neck mass on examination, which feels firm and irregular. On flexible nasendoscopy you note a smooth mass in the left nasal cavity and cannot see beyond the middle meatus. A septal deviation on the right side restricts you from being able to examine the post-nasal space properly due to pain and discomfort. You organise an MRI scan and an ultrasound scan of the neck with tissue sampling. What is the most likely diagnosis in this scenario?
A Olfactory neuroblastoma
B Lymphoma
C Juvenile nasal angiofibroma
D Sarcoma
E Nasopharyngeal carcinoma

24. A 61-year-old man is referred to you from the genitourinary medicine clinic, which he attended for screening after visiting Thailand for a 4-month holiday. He has nasal congestion, dry bloody nasal crusting and blockage symptoms, and admits to using cocaine regularly. On examination he has rhinitis, ulceration and crusting, and you notice a posterior bony septal perforation. Which is the next best step in management?
A Counselling on drug abuse
B Counselling on digital trauma
C ANCA serum blood testing and referral to rheumatology
D Tuberculin skin testing
E Syphilis blood test and penicillin treatment

25. You see a 62-year-old female with left nasal congestion, unilateral epistaxis, with no improvement with saline irrigation. On examination, you visualise a bulky polypoidal mass and are concerned because this clinically appears to be an inverted papilloma. You

schedule her for urgent examination under anaesthesia (EUA) and biopsy. What is the estimated risk of malignant transformation for an inverted papilloma?

A 5%
B 10%
C 15%
D 20%
E 30%

26. You are asked to review a patient from the local orbital MDT. The patient has stable thyroid eye disease, and when they performed a CT scan of the orbits, they noted the patient had an abnormal sphenoid sinus. There is no opacification or evidence of polyposis on the scan. The patient has no sinonasal symptoms. In what percentage of patients does the carotid artery protrude into the sphenoid sinus?

A Less than 10%
B 10–20%
C 20–30%
D 30–40%
E 40–50%

27. A 45-year-old male presents with a history of recurrent epistaxis. He reports that his father also suffered with this same problem. On physical examination you note the lesions pictured in Figure 4.1 and also note the same appearances on the nasal septum, middle turbinate and lateral nasal wall. What is the most likely diagnosis?

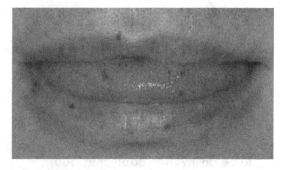

Figure 4.1 Lesions on tongue and lips.

A Haemophilia
B Hereditary haemorrhagic telangiectasia
C Von Willebrand disease
D Neurofibromatosis type 1
E Capillary haemangiomas

28. A 47-year-old female presented to the ENT clinic with nasal blockage, congestion, hyposmia and facial fullness. Flexible nasal endoscopy revealed grade 2 polyps in both nasal cavities and evidence of clear mucin. The post-nasal space was normal. A CT scan reveals a generalised pattern of sinus opacification with polyposis. She is listed for endoscopic sinus surgery to aim to help improve her symptoms and medication delivery. The procedure is undertaken as a routine day case procedure and is uneventful. At follow-up she complains that despite the blockage and obstruction improving, the runny-nose symptom has worsened and is now constant; it is particularly worse when she leans forward. A sample of the nasal liquid is positive for beta-2-transferrin. You request a CT sinus. What is the most likely anatomical site for an injury that could cause her symptoms?

A Posterior table of frontal sinus
B Planum sphenoidale
C Lateral lamella of cribriform plate
D Fovea ethmoidalis
E Clival recess

29. A 44-year-old male comes to see you for follow-up in the rhinology clinic after a CT scan of the sinuses and trial of nasal medications for CRSwNP. The CT scan reveals total opacification of the right and left maxillary sinuses and partial opacification of the right anterior ethmoid air cell with blockage of both osteomeatal complexes (OMC). The other sinuses are clear. What Lund-Mackay score indicates he is a candidate for sinus surgery?

A A score of 5 because a score ≥5 indicates surgical candidacy

B A score of 7 because a score ≥7 indicates surgical candidacy

C A score of 9 because a score ≥9 indicates surgical candidacy

D A score of 12 because a score ≥12 indicates surgical candidacy

E Lund-Mackay is not used to determine surgical candidacy

30. **A 34-year-old male with acute myeloid leukaemia who had a bone-marrow transplant performed 14 days ago was recently admitted for a fever of unknown origin. He is referred by the oncology team with nasal obstruction and headaches. On cranial nerve exam, he reports slight diplopia with extraocular movements. Endoscopy reveals a black right middle turbinate and white hair-like structures on the septum. CT sinuses shows right complete sinus opacification with bony erosion of the posterior maxillary wall and fat stranding of the retroantral fat and masticator space. MRI shows no T2 signal of the mucosa in the maxillary sinus, along the middle turbinate and into the posterior septum travelling up to olfactory cleft. T1 contrast imaging shows lack of dural enhancement in this region. Which of the following factors in his history is not helpful in determining prognosis?**

A An absolute neutrophil could less than 1.0×10^9/L

B Presence of diplopia

C MRI evidence of mucosal dropout and necrosis

D Intracranial spread

E All of the above

31. **You are the on-call ENT consultant and the trauma team calls you for a 21-year-old male who has been assaulted whilst intoxicated. The patient has significant facial injuries and a suspected chest injury. His left eye is swollen shut and there is uncontrollable epistaxis which is difficult to pack due to concerns of a skull base fracture. You have been asked to attend to perform** a lateral canthotomy to temporarily relieve the pressure in the eye. You surmise that the bleeding is most likely from the anterior ethmoidal artery. When considering operative ligation of the anterior ethmoidal artery what is the distance from the anterior lacrimal crest to the foramen of the anterior ethmoidal artery?

A 6 mm

B 12 mm

C 18 mm

D 24 mm

E 30 mm

32. **A 65-year-old man undergoes wide local excision of a basal cell carcinoma from his cheek, leaving behind a defect. The surgeon plans to use a local flap for reconstruction. When considering the width-to-length ratio for the optimal design of a local facial flap, what ratio should be adhered to?**

A 1:1

B 1:2

C 1:3

D 1:4

E 1:5

33. **A 58-year-old male patient had a 1.7 cm squamous cell carcinoma (SCC) on his nasal tip. The lesion was surgically excised, and reconstruction was performed using a paramedian forehead flap. Three weeks post-operatively, while the patient was awaiting the second stage of the flap division and inset, the histopathology report came back, indicating positive margins for the SCC. What is the most appropriate subsequent management plan for this patient?**

A Observe and monitor the patient for any signs of recurrence

B Re-excise the margins to ensure complete removal of the carcinoma

C Proceed with the second stage of flap division and inset without modification

D Initiate adjuvant radiotherapy to the site

E Perform a sentinel lymph node biopsy

34. A 5-year-old child is seen in the emergency department by your registrar with a 2-day history of progressively worsening left periorbital swelling. The child reports eye pain, on a background of a recent viral illness. She has a temperature of 38.4°C and a CRP of 107. Her visual acuity appears intact, the intraocular pressure is normal and there is no evidence of ophthalmoplegia. The CT scan you requested to be performed is concerning for a left subperiosteal abscess. What is the correct Chandler classification for this patient?

A I

B II

C III

D IV

E V

35. A 62-year-old male is referred by his GP with a 2-year history of left nasal obstruction. Nasendoscopy reveals the lesion pictured in Figure 4.2 which is confirmed as inverted papilloma on histopathology. Which virus is most likely to be associated with this pathology?

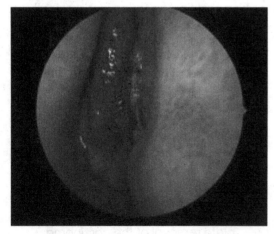

Figure 4.2 Nasal lesion.

A Rhinovirus

B Epstein-Barr virus

C Human papillomavirus

D Herpes zoster virus

E Herpes simplex virus

36. A 47-year-old male is referred to your rhinology clinic with a loss of smell and nasal congestion. He has symptoms of mild rhinitis and denies previous COVID-19 infections. What is the most likely cause of his hyposmia?

A Dementia

B Inflammatory nasal disease

C Head injury

D Malignancy

E Cocaine use

37. A 37-year-old male presents with a 6-month history of progressive right-side nasal obstruction. His sense of smell and taste is normal. He has no nasal discharge. The left side feels normal to him. Endoscopic examination in the clinic reveals a polypoidal lesion filling the right side of the nose. Tissue sampling is concerning for inverted papilloma. CT sinuses show completely opacified right anterior and posterior ethmoid sinuses, a partially opacified right maxillary sinus with hyperostosis of the bone on the posterior maxillary wall, a right sphenoid sinus without disease and a right frontal sinus with a fluid level and frothy secretions. There is septal deviation to the left and the left-sided sinuses are without any mucosal disease. What is the most likely site of origin of the inverted papilloma based on these CT findings?

A Ethmoid sinus because it is completely opacified

B Frontal sinus because it shows evidence of fluid secretions and inverted papilloma are highly secretory

C Maxillary sinus because of the hyperostosis of posterior maxillary wall

D Lateral nasal wall because the sphenoid sinus is not involved with any disease

E Septum given the septal deviation

38. You are referred a 41-year-old invest-ment banker for review, who presents with nasal congestion, whistling and crusting as seen in Figure 4.3. He is otherwise well and denies using rec-reational drugs or previous sinonasal surgery. What is the best initial therapy for this patient?

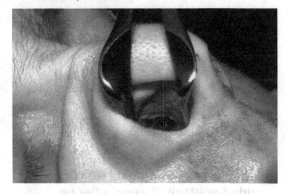

Figure 4.3 Nostril.

   A Surgical removal of crusting and divi-sion of adhesions
   B Surgical repair of the septal perfora-tion using advancement flaps
   C Silastic septal button
   D Biopsy of the septal perforation
   E Nasal douching and nasal creams/emollients

39. An 80-year-old male on anticoagula-tion for a metallic heart valve presents with significant epistaxis that is non-responsive to initial management. Given his complex medical back-ground, he is not considered a suitable candidate for general anaesthesia and operative intervention. Which of the fol-lowing vessels should not routinely be embolised in patients with epistaxis?
   A Anterior ethmoid artery
   B Palatovaginal artery
   C Facial artery
   D Internal maxillary artery
   E Sphenopalatine

40. A 22-year-old female presents with a 2-year history of chronic rhinitis.

She has had intermittent symptoms of congestion and rhinorrhoea, and reports worsening severity of symptoms to cold, dry air. She has not had much benefit with topical nasal steroid trials. Allergy testing and cross-sectional imaging were unremarkable. She is otherwise fit and well, with no medi-cal allergies. What is the mechanism of action for the medication that is most appropriate for her treatment?
   A Blocking release of histamine
   B Blocking adrenergic receptors
   C Blocking nicotinic receptors
   D Blocking cholinergic receptors
   E Stabilising mast cell membranes

41. What is the appropriate excision mar-gin for a melanoma with a depth of 1–2 mm located on the face?
   A 5 mm margin
   B 1 cm margin
   C 1 to 2 cm margin
   D 2 to 3 cm margin
   E 3 cm margin

42. A Z-plasty can be used to lengthen a contracted scar. Which of these Z-angles is correctly paired with the length gained from the Z-plasty?
   A 30 degrees – 30%
   B 45 degrees – 60%
   C 60 degrees – 75%
   D 70 degrees – 75%
   E 90 degrees – 90%

43. A 30-year-old tennis player with aller-gic rhinitis secondary to grass contin-ues to have ongoing nasal congestion despite treatment with fluticasone nasal spray. Which of the following additional medications is most likely to help improve his symptoms?
   A Montelukast tablet once daily
   B Sodium cromoglycate eyedrops twice daily
   C Cetirizine tablet once daily
   D Beclomethasone inhaler twice daily
   E Azelastine nasal spray twice daily

44. You review a 47-year-old female who has chronic rhinosinusitis with nasal polyps, asthma and an allergic reaction to aspirin. She has had multiple sinus surgeries and has been compliant with maximal topical therapy, but her polyps have shown regrowth worsening subjective symptoms. You refer her to your immunology colleague for consideration of aspirin desensitisation or biological therapies. Which of these statements is correct?

    A Biological therapies are ineffective in treating aspirin-exacerbated respiratory disease (AERD)

    B Biological therapies for AERD are only effective after sinus surgery

    C Dupilumab (Dupixent) is an IL-5 and IL-13 blocking monoclonal antibody

    D Aspirin desensitisation is most effective if administered after sinus surgery

    E Aspirin desensitisation reduces the size of existing polyps

45. A 42-year-old tennis coach is referred via their GP to your outpatient clinic with a 5-year history of pruritis, sneezing and nasal congestion during summer. They are otherwise fit and well, with no history of previous sinonasal surgery. They have declined topical therapy due to concerns around potential side effects. Flexible nasendoscopy demonstrates diffuse mucosal oedema throughout the nose with cobblestoning, bilateral bluish-grey inferior turbinates and clear mucin within the nasal cavity. What is the most appropriate initial medical management?

    A Intranasal antihistamine

    B Oral antihistamine

    C Intranasal steroid

    D Oral steroid

    E Aerosolised steroid (inhaler)

46. A 79-year-old male presents to your outpatient clinic with a 4-month history of unilateral nasal congestion. Head and neck examination is unremarkable, but flexible nasendoscopy demonstrates a suspicious right-sided nasopharyngeal mass arising from the fossa of Rosenmuller. What other findings are you likely to encounter?

    A Ipsilateral palatal immobility, glue ear and trigeminal neuralgia

    B Ipsilateral hypoglossal nerve palsy, abducens nerve palsy and trigeminal neuralgia

    C Ipsilateral palatal immobility, hypoglossal nerve palsy and glue ear

    D Ipsilateral glue ear, trigeminal neuralgia and facial nerve palsy

    E Ipsilateral ptosis, miosis and enophthalmos

47. A 43-year-old male presents to the emergency department with right-sided epistaxis, 2 weeks after an external dacryocystorhinostomy (DCR). What would be the next most appropriate surgical intervention for this patient should conservative measures be unsuccessful?

    A Right external anterior ethmoidal artery ligation

    B Right endoscopic anterior ethmoidal artery ligation

    C Right endoscopic sphenopalatine artery ligation

    D Embolisation of the right sphenopalatine artery

    E Right external carotid artery ligation

48. A 62-year-old male presents to your anosmia clinic, with olfactory disturbance present for 18 months following a COVID-19 infection. He is assessed using the University of Pennsylvania smell identification test (UPSIT). Which of the following scores is suggestive of malingering?

    A <5

    B <8

    C <10

    D <12

    E <14

49. A 25-year-old male presents to the ED after sustaining a facial injury in a physical altercation. He complains of pain in the maxillary region, and on examination, you note mobility of the upper teeth. His eye region and forehead are intact with no visible deformities or palpable steps. Based on these findings, which of the following fractures is most likely?
    A LeFort 1 fracture
    B LeFort 2 fracture
    C LeFort 3 fracture
    D Orbital blowout fracture
    E Zygomatic arch fracture

50. A 45-year-old man is involved in a bicycle accident and is thrown into a barbed-wire fence. He suffers an avulsion of approximately 50% of his upper lip with loss of the amputated part. Subsequently he undergoes reconstruction of his upper lip defect using an Abbe flap with a lower lip donor site. At what time point post-operatively is the flap typically divided?
    A 7 days
    B 10 days
    C 21 days
    D 28 days
    E 35 days

51. An 82-year-old male presents with a slow growing non-distinct lesion over his right alar cartilage. A punch biopsy demonstrates a morphoeic basal cell carcinoma. What is the most appropriate step in his management?
    A 4 mm margin with full thickness skin graft
    B 8 mm margin with a bilobed flap
    C 1 cm margin with delayed reconstruction
    D 13 mm margin with primary closure
    E Referral to local Mohs service

52. Basal cell carcinoma (BCC) can manifest in various clinical and histological subtypes. Which subtype is characterised by a central ulcer with raised pearly edges?
    A Superficial BCC
    B Nodular BCC
    C Infiltrative BCC
    D Morpheaform (sclerosing) BCC
    E Pigmented BCC

53. Lentigo maligna is a subtype of melanoma that primarily occurs on sun-exposed areas of the skin, such as the face. Which characteristic feature is commonly associated with lentigo maligna?
    A Rapid growth and metastasis
    B Presence of keratin pearls
    C Radial growth phase
    D Irregular borders with various colours
    E Extensive in situ growth and atypical melanocytes

54. A 43-year-old female presents with right-sided clear nasal discharge. Fluid sampling confirms the presence of beta-2-transferrin. A high-resolution CT sinus fails to localise the site of a potential defect. What would be the next most appropriate step in management?
    A Endoscopic exploration and repair
    B Intrathecal fluorescein and assessment in clinic
    C T2-weighted MRI with CISS/FIESTA sequence
    D CT cisternography
    E Acetazolamide 250 mg TDS and clinic review in 6 weeks

55. The superior turbinate is used as an anatomical landmark in sinus surgery. Which ethmoturbinal is it derived from?
    A First
    B Second
    C Third
    D Fourth
    E Fifth

56. A 47-year-old female is postop day 5 following vestibular schwannoma resection via a retrosigmoid

approach. The neurotologist states that the facial nerve is anatomically intact but the nerve could not be stimulated at the brainstem following tumour resection. On physical exam, the patient has complete ipsilateral facial paralysis. The best long-term course of action regarding corneal protection is:

A Eye care only with artificial tears, Lacri-Lube and nighttime taping
B Placement of gold weight
C Tarsal strip procedure
D Combined tarsal strip and gold weight
E Eye taping day and night for 2 weeks

57. **What is the time limit that will allow the surgeon to utilise the nerve stimulator intraoperatively to assist in identification of distal branches of a severed facial nerve?**

A 12 hours
B 24 hours
C 36 hours
D 48 hours
E 72 hours

58. **You are undertaking a bilateral functional endoscopic sinus surgery (FESS) for CRSwNP and enter the posterior ethmoids through the basal lamella. Which of the following is NOT one of the constant Messerklinger landmarks?**

A Uncinate process
B Face of bulla
C Basal lamella of middle turbinate
D Superior turbinate basal lamella
E Face of sphenoid

59. **A 55-year-old female has been diagnosed with an ivory osteoma of the right frontal sinus. During functional endoscopic sinus surgery, your trainee asks about access to the frontal sinus. Which of the following is not a boundary of the frontal recess?**

A Middle turbinate
B Face of bulla

C Agger nasi
D Lamina papyracea
E Ascending process of maxilla

60. **You are called to review a patient 10 minutes following the completion of bilateral FESS surgery. The patient has epistaxis and severe left orbital pain, with visible left periorbital ecchymosis and a tense globe on palpation. You are unable to open the eye to examine further. What is the most appropriate subsequent management of this patient?**

A Tonometry
B Intravenous acetazolamide
C Intravenous dexamethasone
D Lateral canthotomy and cantholysis
E Pack nasal cavity and arrange urgent ophthalmology review

61. **A 19-year-old female with a 2-week history of worsening headaches presents to the emergency department with a reduced GCS. Cross sectional imaging by CT and MRI confirms complete opacification of the left maxillary, ethmoid, sphenoid and frontal sinuses, with a frontal empyema. The neurosurgical consultant plans to undertake a craniotomy and evacuation of the empyema. What is the most appropriate surgical intervention for the frontal sinus?**

A Modified Lothrop procedure
B Frontal sinus trephine
C Endoscopic Draf 2a
D No surgical intervention warranted. Offer medical management with nasal steroids, decongestant and antibiotics
E Limited FESS and observation

62. **A 15-year-old male presents with presentation of progressive bilateral nasal obstruction. On flexible endoscopy you note a bilateral nasopharyngeal mass filling the left nasal cavity. MRI shows a highly vascular tumour filling**

the nasopharynx, tracking into the left pterygopalatine fossa with anterior displacement of the left posterior maxillary wall. Prior to surgical resection an angiogram was performed by your interventional radiology colleagues and bilateral embolisation of his internal maxillary arteries was performed with complete reduction of flow through both arteries feeding the tumour. During surgery the following day, profuse bleeding was encountered near the sphenoid rostrum bilaterally and he required transfusion of 4 units of packed red blood cells. What artery was likely contributing to this complication?

A Vidian
B Sphenopalatine
C Pharyngeal
D Descending palatine
E Inferior turbinate

63. A 45-year-old male presents to your outpatient clinic for the results of his CT and MRI scan, after being reviewed by your registrar with a 12-month history of an infero-laterally displaced right globe. He has no changes in his vision. His past medical history was unremarkable except for a previous road traffic accident at age 30. Cross-sectional imaging demonstrated a homogenous high signal on T2-weighted MRI and low signal on T1-weighted MRI, with CT demonstrating an opacified right frontal sinus, with an expansile lesion and posterior table erosion. What is the best first course of management?

A Endoscopic sinus surgery with biopsy or marsupialisation/decompression
B Endoscopic resection and skull base reconstruction with nasoseptal flap
C Bicoronal incision, osteoplastic flap and cranialisation of frontal sinus with neurosurgery assistance.

D Urgent trephination and drainage
E Antibiotics and a course of oral steroids

64. A 33-year-old male presents to your clinic with features of severe rhinitis. You offer to prescribe topical steroid therapy, but he is reluctant given the associated risks. He asks about the range of topical therapies available and their systemic absorption. Which of the following statements is incorrect?

A Fluticasone: 0.5% systemic absorption
B Mometasone: 0.5% systemic absorption
C Budesonide: 33% systemic absorption
D Beclomethasone: 55% systemic absorption
E Betamethasone: 100% systemic absorption

65. During an endoscopic endonasal hypophysectomy, a medical student asks about the anatomy of the internal carotid artery system. Which of the following statements is incorrect regarding the Cincinnati classification of internal carotid artery segments?

A C1: Cervical
B C3: Lacerum
C C5: Cavernous
D C6: Ophthalmic
E C7: Communicating

66. A 62-year-old female presents with left-sided nasal congestion and malar discomfort. Endoscopy demonstrates a polypoidal mass, and a local anaesthetic biopsy is undertaken in clinic, which confirms your suspicion of an inverted papilloma. Her resultant CT scan is shown in Figure 4.4. What grade on the Krouse classification of sinonasal inverted papilloma does the patient fit?

A 1
B 2
C 3

D 4

E 5

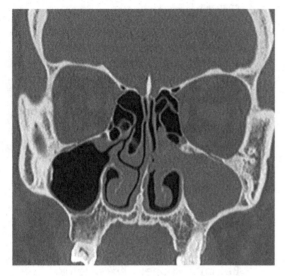

Figure 4.4 CT scan.

67. **During a local anaesthetic skin surgery list, the medical student asks what the most superficial layer of the epidermis is.**
    A Stratum basale
    B Stratum corneum
    C Stratum lucidum
    D Stratum spinosum
    E Stratum granulosum

68. **A 49-year-old otherwise fit and well individual presents with double vision and nasal congestion. Clinical examination reveals a failure in abduction of the left eye, but no palpable lymphadenopathy. Flexible nasendoscopy demonstrates a large mass within the nasopharynx with retained secretions. A biopsy is undertaken under a local anaesthetic, and cross-sectional imaging with a CT and MRI requested. Histology is reported as containing physaliphorous cells. Which of the following statements regarding the pathology is incorrect?**
    A They are found most commonly in the clivus within the spheno-occipital sub-group

B On cross-sectional imaging they are usually found off the midline
C Are characterised by intratumoural calcification
D Metastatic spread is rare
E Mainstay of treatment is surgical resection and post-operative radiotherapy

69. **A 32-year-old female model presents to your clinic with nasal obstruction following nasal trauma. On examination she has a C-shaped nasal deformity, with poor tip support secondary to a short caudal septum. She is under-rotated with a nasolabial angle of 80 degrees. Endoscopic examination reveals a high anterior septal deflection to the right with a left inferior maxillary crest spur. She has agreed to proceed with an open septorhinoplasty. At the end of the procedure you turn your attention to addressing her under-rotated tip. Which of the following methods is NOT likely to address this aspect?**
    A Columellar strut graft
    B Lateral crural steal
    C Ansa graft
    D Medial crural reduction
    E Septal extension graft

70. **A 47-year-old male presents to your clinic with a long history of left frontal headaches. Flexible nasendoscopy is unremarkable. You request a CT scan of his paranasal sinuses, which demonstrates the findings in Figure 4.5. Which of the following statements regarding the findings and likely pathology is INCORRECT?**
    A It is most commonly found within the ethmoid sinuses
    B It is the most common neoplasm of the paranasal sinuses
    C It usually has a male predominance
    D It is often found within the fourth decade
    E It can be associated with Gardner syndrome

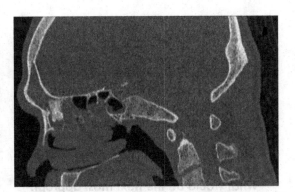

Figure 4.5 CT scan.

71. **A 60-year-old man with histologically proven melanoma of his cheek is discussed at the skin cancer MDT. In the management of melanoma, what is the primary purpose of a sentinel lymph node biopsy?**
    A To confirm the diagnosis of melanoma
    B To determine the melanoma's depth of invasion
    C To assess the presence of distant metastasis
    D To identify the first regional lymph node(s) at risk of metastasis
    E To guide the choice of systemic chemotherapy

72. **A 63-year-old man presents with a skin lesion on the side wall of his nose and a long history of sun exposure. In the clinical examination of a skin lesion suspected of being either a basal cell carcinoma (BCC) or a squamous cell carcinoma (SCC), which characteristic is more commonly associated with BCC?**
    A Rapid growth
    B Ulceration
    C Central crusting
    D Pearly or translucent appearance
    E Reddish coloration

73. **During a bilateral FESS, your attention turns to addressing the frontal sinuses with a right-sided Draf 2a procedure. During instrumentation, you notice a CSF leak, and widen access with an axillectomy. You note a small 2 mm**

defect superiorly in the posterior table. **Which of the following is the most appropriate next step in the management of this patient?**
    A A nasoseptal flap overlay, Surgicel and Tisseel
    B Inferior turbinate flap overlay, Surgicel and Tisseel
    C Pericranial flap
    D Free mucosal overlay, Surgicel and Tisseel
    E IV antibiotics, bed rest and lumbar drain for 3 days

74. **You review the CT scan of a 33-year-old female who presented with bilateral nasal polyps. She has a Lund-Mackay score of 24/24, and the report mentions the possibility of fungal colonisation. Which of the following is not one of the Bent and Kuhn criteria for allergic fungal rhinosinusitis?**
    A Mixed density sign on imaging
    B Presence of non-invasive fungal hyphae
    C Polyposis
    D Type 2 hypersensitivity
    E Eosinophilic mucin

75. **An 81-year-old male presents to you with a 4-month history of a lesion over his right forehead. Head and neck examination is otherwise unremarkable. A 4 mm punch biopsy is undertaken in clinic, and histology confirms a squamous cell carcinoma (SCC). Which of the following features is not a high-risk feature of a cutaneous SCC?**
    A Immunosuppression
    B Clark level ≥4
    C 1 mm depth of invasion
    D >2 cm tumour diameter
    E Perineural invasion

76. **A 24-year-old male presents to your clinic with anosmia, nasal congestion and visual disturbances. Head and neck examination is unremarkable. Flexible nasendoscopy confirms a large mass arising within the right**

olfactory cleft. Ophthalmology review confirms right-sided papilloedema and left optic atrophy. Combination imaging of CT/MRI showed a dumbbell-shaped mass breaching the skull base and compressing both frontal lobes with vasogenic oedema. A biopsy of the tumour is taken in clinic and is reported as showing small round blue cell morphology. Of the following which pathology can be excluded from the differential diagnosis?

A Melanoma

B Rhabdomyosarcoma

C Sinonasal undifferentiated carcinoma

D Esthesioneuroblastoma

E Adenocarcinoma

77. Which one of the following is not considered a risk factor for spontaneous cerebrospinal fluid leaks of the anterior skull base?

A Venous sinus thrombosis

B Female sex

C Elevated BMI

D Idiopathic intracranial hypertension

E Hypertension

78. A 78-year-old female presents with diplopia and was found to have a right sixth nerve palsy. MRI of the skull base identified a clival lesion extending to the petroclival junction which was hyperintense on T1 and T2. Radiologically this was consistent with a chondrosarcoma, and an endoscopic excision was planned. A post-operative MRI showed a significant debulk with likely small volume residual tumour laterally in the petrous apex medial to the great vessels. What would be the most appropriate subsequent management?

A Further endoscopic excision

B Middle cranial fossa approach for excision of residuum

C Stereotactic radiotherapy

D Proton beam therapy

E Watch and wait

79. A 27-year-old female presents with a large left-sided aggressive orbital mass and was found to be 26 weeks pregnant. She has significant retro-orbital pain and severe proptosis with rapid visual decline over 24 hours. An MRI shows an intra-orbital mass extending into the ethmoid and frontal sinuses. What would be the next most appropriate management strategy?

A Local anaesthetic endonasal biopsy and await histology

B General anaesthetic biopsy and maximal debulk of tumour to preserve vision

C Local anaesthetic external biopsy

D Admit and treat with IV steroids

E General anaesthetic biopsy and await histology

80. A 70-year-old male presents with headaches and is found to have bitemporal hemianopia. An MRI demonstrates a pituitary macroadenoma, which is non-functioning on hormonal assay. The report further states that the tumour is extending into the right cavernous sinus and extending above the intra-cavernous carotid artery in the superior cavernous sinus (Knosp grade 3A). Which cranial nerve(s) is/are most at risk from this tumour?

A Olfactory nerves

B Abducens nerve

C Oculomotor and trochlear nerves

D Oculomotor nerve

E Trigeminal nerve

81. You are reviewing a 60-year-old man who has recently immigrated from Bangladesh. He shows you a raised lesion on his nose which is consistent with a basal cell carcinoma. He tells you that he has similar lesions on his chest. When you examine him you note that he has keratosis of his palms and white lines in his nails. To which

heavy metal has he likely had chronic exposure?

A Arsenic
B Manganese
C Chromium
D Lead
E Cadmium

82. You are reviewing a 64-year-old female in clinic. Recently you saw her to perform a wide local excision of a 2 cm flesh-coloured, scar-like plaque on her cheek. The pathology result is not available in the clinical notes, so you decide to call the pathologist. The pathologist tells you that the lesion is a basal cell carcinoma and that it is showing deep invasion. You recognise from the location of the lesion that this was at an embryonic fusion plane. Which BCC subtype is most likely?

A Morpheaform
B Nodular
C Superficial
D Fibroepithelial
E Micronodular

83. A 45-year-old patient is diagnosed with a squamous cell carcinoma of the external nose. You are discussing the potential pathways for lymphatic spread with a colleague. Which cervical lymph node level is most directly involved in the primary drainage of the external nose?

A Level IA
B Level IB
C Level II
D Level III
E Level IV

84. A 6-year-old child is brought to your clinic by her parents for follow-up. The child underwent repair of a unilateral cleft lip and palate during infancy. They express concerns regarding her facial appearance because she is about to

start school. On examination, you note a well-healed scar on the upper lip, asymmetry of the nostrils, and a significantly short columella, which is the parents' primary concern. Which of the surgical techniques is commonly used to address a shortened columella in this scenario?

A Z-plasty
B Rhomboid flap
C V-Y advancement flap
D Abbe flap
E Bilobed flap

85. You are called by the emergency department (ED) for advice on the management of a 26-year-old man who has been in a bike accident and sustained a laceration to his nose. The ED doctor is concerned that there is exposure of the nasal bone. Given the anatomically variable thickness of the nasal skin, where are the nasal bones most likely exposed?

A Glabella
B Columella
C Rhinion
D Nasion
E Radix

86. A 55-year-old woman presents to the ED 48 hours post rhytidectomy with a facial haematoma. On examination, you note a tense, swollen area measuring approximately 4 cm in diameter. What is the most appropriate immediate step in management?

A Prescribe oral antibiotics
B Advise cold compress and observation
C Schedule an outpatient follow-up in one week
D Take the patient back to theatre for evacuation
E Administer intravenous steroids

87. A 62-year-old man presents with a longstanding history of nasal

enlargement and thickened, reddened nasal skin. The surface appears nodular and is accompanied by large pores. Based on the clinical diagnosis of rhinophyma, you discuss management options with him. Which of the following treatments provides the best cosmetic outcome for this condition?

A Topical metronidazole
B Oral antibiotics
C Cryotherapy
D Dermabrasion
E Intralesional steroids

88. A 28-year-old woman presents to the emergency department following a motor vehicle accident. On examination, you note significant facial swelling, bilateral periorbital ecchymosis and an increased intercanthal distance. The nasal bridge appears widened and flattened. There is a clear fluid dripping from her nose. Which of the following fractures is most likely responsible for her presentation?

A LeFort II fracture
B Zygomaticomaxillary complex fracture
C Orbital blowout fracture
D Nasoethmoidal fracture
E Frontal bone fracture

89. A 58-year-old woman presents with complaints of upper eyelid drooping, making her appear tired and mildly obstructing her vision. After a thorough evaluation, a decision is made to proceed with an upper blepharoplasty. When performing this procedure, what is the typical maximum amount of skin that is safely removed from the upper eyelid to avoid complications?

A 2–4 mm
B 5–7 mm
C 8–10 mm
D 11–13 mm
E 14–16 mm

90. A 16-year-old boy is scheduled for a pinnaplasty for his prominent ears. The surgeon is describing the surgical technique to his registrar. He plans to use a technique that primarily involves post-auricular skin excision and placing mattress sutures to recreate the antihelical fold. Which surgical technique is being described?

A Stenström technique
B Furnas technique
C Converse technique
D Mustardé technique
E Davis technique

91. A 52-year-old woman presents to clinic with a 3-month history of painful oral ulcers. She has been avoiding food due to pain and has lost 4 kg. Recently, she noticed some fluid-filled blisters on her chest, back and face. These blisters are soft to touch, and some have spontaneously ruptured, leaving behind raw areas. She also mentions that when she tries to burst the blisters by pressing a finger alongside them, they seem to extend further. Histopathology from one of the blisters shows intraepidermal blistering due to acantholysis. Which of the following conditions is the patient most likely suffering from?

A Bullous impetigo
B Bullous pemphigoid
C Pemphigus vulgaris
D Erythema multiforme
E Stevens-Johnson syndrome

92. A 58-year-old man undergoes Mohs surgery to a 1 cm lesion on the nasal tip that undergoes a skin graft reconstruction. He comes back to see you 3 years later and tells you that he is suffering severe shooting pains from the excision site. Examination shows a well healed surgical site with no signs of recurrence. It is likely he is suffering from neuralgia originating from which nerve?

A Supratrochlear nerve (V1 branch)

B Infratrochlear nerve (V1 branch)
C External branch of anterior ethmoid nerve (V1 branch)
D Infraorbital nerve (V2 branch)
E Mental nerve (V3 branch)

93. A 74-year-old female requires excision of a 1cm lesion on her cheek. The lesion appears pearly with central depression and a rolled border. What is the recommended margin to achieve complete removal while optimising cosmetic outcomes?
A 1 mm
B 2 mm
C 3 mm
D 4 mm
E 5 mm

94. A 56-year-old female presents with an asymmetric pigmented lesion on her neck. Which of the following is an essential step to assess the characteristics of the lesion and determine the need for treatment?
A Direct excision of the lesion
B Clinical observation without intervention
C Dermoscopy examination
D Punch biopsy of the lesion
E Sentinel lymph node biopsy

95. A 64-year-old man presents with a lesion measuring approximately 3 mm on the helical rim that has been present for 6 months and does not appear to be growing. It is exquisitely tender to touch but not painful at other times. What is the most common predisposing factor associated with the likely cause?
A Excessive sun exposure
B Bacterial infection
C Autoimmune disorder
D Trauma or pressure
E Genetic mutation

96. Uptake failure following full-thickness skin graft is most often secondary to which complication?

A Local fluid collection underlying graft
B Graft mobility
C Excessive graft thickness
D Recipient site devascularisation
E Graft donor site infection

97. A 65-year-old heavy smoker, with diabetes, with a large, near-total cutaneous dorsal/tip nasal defect presents for closure following a Mohs resection for squamous cell carcinoma. On exam, you note a low anterior hairline. Which is the best choice in reconstructive options?
A Paramedian forehead flap – two stage
B Midline forehead flap – two stage
C Paramedian forehead flap – three stage
D Midline forehead flap – three stage
E Full thickness skin graft

98. During an endoscopic hypophysectomy for a non-functioning macroadenoma, with suprasellar extension, you experience a moderate CSF leak, and find a small defect within the diaphragma sellae. This is addressed with abdominal fat, and a free-mucosal graft. Prior to closure of the defect, what grade is the leak according to the most commonly cited grading scale?
A Grade 0
B Grade 1
C Grade 2
D Grade 3
E Grade 4

99. The frontal (temporal) branch of the facial nerve is at risk when harvesting a temporoparietal fascia flap. Which best describes the course of the frontal branch?
A Follows a line from the external auditory canal to the superolateral orbital rim
B Follows a line from 0.5 cm below the tragus to 1.5 cm above the lateral brow

C Travels subcutaneously superior to the zygomatic arch

D Crosses the zygomatic arch in the anterior third

E Travels superior 3 cm anterior to the tragus

100. **Nasal decongestants aid airflow through vasoconstriction of nasal vasculature.**

Which neurotransmitter is relevant when considering the most commonly available over-the-counter medications?

A Serotonin

B Adrenaline

C Acetylcholine

D Glutamate

E Dopamine

ANSWERS

1. **Answer D**

   The history and findings are consistent with a spontaneous CSF leak likely due to idiopathic intracranial hypertension (IIH). Neuro-ophthalmology plays a crucial role in diagnosis because they are able to perform a detailed ocular assessment, specifically examining the fundus for evidence of papilloedema. In IIH visual field defects are more common than problems with visual acuity. Patients often present late due to the slow development of the visual deficit which allows compensation. Visual field defects in IIH are a direct result of changes in the optic nerve, specifically the optic nerve head. This is most likely due to changes in the autoregulation and microcirculation of the optic disc. In IIH the most common and frequently occurring visual field defect is an enlargement of the blind spot. Other visual field defects that can occur are like defects found in glaucoma:
   - Generalised constriction
   - Loss of nasal visual fields (particularly inferonasal)
   - Arcuate defects
   - Scotomas

2. **Answer B**

   In CRSsNP type two disease (chronic rhinosinusitis without nasal polyps) that does not respond to topical nasal rinsing and nasal steroid therapy, EPOS 2020 recommends a 3-month course of a macrolide antibiotic such as clarithromycin. ECG assessment is imperative, since in patients with long QT syndrome, cardiac disease or patients taking other QT prolonging medications, clarithromycin can provoke life-threatening arrhythmias.

3. **Answer E**

   This patient has had a traumatic nasal injury and subsequently has bilateral nasal obstruction, with a structural external deformity. An external septorhinoplasty is the most appropriate procedure because with a C-shaped deformity, the middle third of the nose is involved and this is most often addressed with an external approach. A positive Cottle's manoeuvre is indicative of internal nasal valve collapse, which is addressed using spreader grafts. Whilst alar collapse may be related to a severe septal deformity and altered nasal flow dynamics, it is reasonable to assume that an alar batten graft is warranted.

4. **Answer C**

   This type of deformity can often arise when the upper lateral cartilages are not reattached to the septum during an external septorhinoplasty. During a bony/cartilaginous dorsal resection or de-hump, the spreader mechanism of the 'T-frame' of the nose is disrupted and impacts the stabilisation of the upper lateral cartilages, resulting in them becoming free-floating. It is this separation, and movement over time, that leads to an inverted V deformity. When separated, they can migrate to a posterior, medial and cranial position relative to the nasal bones.

5. **Answer C**

    Despite cocaine prevalence rising within the UK, and septal surgery being a known risk factor for septal perforation, the most common cause is still due to digital or local trauma. It is important when approaching patients with a septal perforation to take a thorough but delicate history questioning digital trauma, cocaine use, previous surgery and family or individual risk factors for granulomatous disease, including systemic symptoms. Performing screening bloods for FBC, renal function, ACE and calcium, ANCA and PR3/MPO are helpful in the diagnostic work-up to ensure you do not miss an underlying systemic condition, though these may also be raised in cocaine use. Performing urine screening for substance misuse is also crucial, since patients sometimes may be reluctant to admit to using illicit drugs.

6. **Answer D**

    The maxillary nerve (V2) is the second division of the trigeminal nerve and most at risk here because it passes through the foramen rotundum in the pterygopalatine fossa (PPF). The nerve exits the PPF in several branches to innervate the face and nasal cavity but one branch, the infraorbital nerve, exits superiorly along the roof of the maxillary sinus.

    The maxillary nerve has both sensory and motor functions and iatrogenic injury to the maxillary nerve can occur with surgery to this region and can lead to hypoaethesia/numbness over the cheek or mid-face or even severe neuropathic type pain, as seen in trigeminal neuralgia.

7. **Answer C**

    A Pott's puffy tumour is a subperiosteal abscess due to associated frontal skull osteomyelitis. This usually occurs as a rare complication of frontal sinusitis or trauma to the forehead that presents with tender forehead swelling associated with fever, headaches, nasal discharge or meningism. Osteomyelitis can occur due to haematogenous spread of the infection or due to direct extension of infection through immature sinuses/bone. Although the most common cause of Pott's puffy tumour is polymicrobial (streptococci, anaerobes and staphylococci) bacterium, non-enterococci streptococci are the most prevalent, present in almost 50% of cases. In the presence of intracranial spread, the most common organism is *Streptococcus milleri*. Management includes a combination of medical treatment with broad spectrum systemic antibiotics (until microbiology results can tailor specific treatment) and surgical treatment. The length of medical therapy is governed by intracranial spread, and if present, is usually for a duration of 1–12 weeks. Immediate surgical intervention is in the form of drainage of the abscess and frontal sinus washout with a trephine. Sinus surgery is likely to be complicated by severe inflammation and bleeding and should be reserved for an elective setting (functional endoscopic sinus surgery [FESS] and Draf sinusotomy).

8. **Answer B**

    When managing inferior turbinate hypertrophy medical management should always be employed before pursuing surgical correction. Topical steroids are often the most effective therapy in controlling nasal obstruction related to inferior turbinate hypertrophy and topical antihistamines are useful in patients with allergy-proven allergic rhinitis. Oral antihistamines are often helpful for the symptom constellation of allergic rhinitis, but not as effective as topical therapy, and systemic treatment has more side effects. Subcutaneous immunotherapy is a good option to help reduce the symptoms of allergic rhinitis but not a requirement to offer surgery and the patient should be informed that this is an option in treatment and can be referred to an allergist to discuss the cost and benefits of this type of therapy. Serum IgE levels will enable assessment of the allergic component of his symptoms and the tailoring of his medication and treatment plan but are not effective in surgical decision making.

9. **Answer D**

Although risk factors for OSA vary and being male and having a high BMI and large neck circumference (collar size exceeding 17) are common findings, severe OSA is most commonly associated with hypertension – which itself can result in elevated long-term cardiovascular risk if left untreated. Other findings include a bradycardia. A detailed history to exclude apnoeic episodes, and daytime somnolence should be taken, with DVLA notification imperative by law, if any OSA features are present. An Epworth sleepiness score, although not diagnostic, will provide a clinician with a probability of OSA. Any patient with features of OSA should be referred to their local respiratory team for sleep studies.

10. **Answer D**

Beta-2-transferrin, previously known as tau protein, is produced by the activity of neuraminidase on transferrin. It is found only in the CSF, the aqueous humour of the eye and the perilymph. It has a reported 70–100% sensitivity and specificity for detecting CSF. Rare transferrin allelic variants, chronic liver disease and alcoholism may cause false positive results, and comparison of serum and CSF may be required to rule out these false positives.

11. **Answer C**

The internal nasal valve is the narrowest part of the nasal airway and is formed by the junction of the septum, upper lateral cartilage and inferior turbinate. In Caucasians the ideal angle of the internal nasal valve ranges from 10° to 15° and accounts for approximately 50% of the nasal resistance.

Spreader grafts are rectangular septal cartilaginous grafts positioned between the dorsal aspect of the septum and the upper lateral cartilages. They are particularly useful for supporting the internal nasal valve, widening the piriform aperture and straightening a deviated septum. In cases in which there is a compromised or narrowed internal nasal valve, such as this patient, spreader grafts act to open this area and facilitate airflow.

The other options have various purposes:

- Alar batten grafts: Reinforce the lateral nasal wall to treat or prevent external valve collapse.
- Caudal septal extension graft: Influence the position and shape of the nasal tip. It can be used to provide projection, rotation, or support to the tip.
- Columellar strut: Designed to support and stabilise the nasal tip. It can be beneficial in cases in which there is a lack of tip support.
- Butterfly graft: Unlike spreader grafts these are harvested from the auricular cartilage. They are onlay grafts placed dorsally between the septum and upper lateral cartilages. Additional risk of donor site morbidity and occasional widening of the supratip area with fullness in the middle third of the nose means these grafts are less frequently used than spreader grafts.

12. Answer A

The sensory innervation to the external ear originates from both cranial and spinal nerves, specifically, branches of the cranial nerves V (auriculotemporal), VII (nervus intermedius), X (auricular branch of the vagus), and the lesser occipital (C2, C3) and greater auricular nerve (C2, C3) nerves. During facelift procedures, the greater auricular nerve is the most commonly injured nerve. The nerve is divided into an anterior and posterior branch. The anterior branch is distributed to the skin over parotid gland and angle of mandible. The posterior branch innervates the skin over the mastoid, the lower posterior pinna, the lobule and the lower concha. The nerve is most vulnerable at the root of the helix during raising of skin flaps, where it may lie superficially. It may also be injured during time of posterior platysmal suspension. The majority of rhytidectomy patients will have transient paraesthesia due to transection of smaller sensory nerves, but the transection of the greater auricular nerve may result in more significant symptoms including painful neuromas, pain with cold exposure and neuralgia/dysesthesia.

13. Answer C

Rhinoscleroma is a chronic granulomatous disease primarily of the nose but with potential involvement of the rest of the upper respiratory tract. It is caused by infection with *Klebsiella rhinoscleromatis*, a Gram negative *Klebsiella pneumoniae* subspecies. It affects women more than men (1.6:1), and is endemic to Egypt, Indonesia and Central America. The best imaging modality to assess disease extent is a T1 MRI with contrast, whereby you would expect to see a high T1 intensity signal due to increased protein content within Mikulicz cells and Russell bodies, and inhomogeneous contrast enhancement in areas of fibrosis. The MRI scan can provide a triplanar view of disease extension and invasion into local anatomical structures. Management includes nasal rinsing, topical nasal steroids and oral tetracycline antibiotics. Tissue sampling is crucial to confirm the diagnosis since nasal swabs are often not diagnostic. This disease can cause significant scarring and crusting throughout the nasal cavity.

14. Answer C

A known complication of orbital cellulitis is cavernous sinus thrombosis. This is particularly of concern in those who are immunocompromised, as in this clinical scenario. Progression of infection in these patients can be rapid, mandating regular clinical review. Clinical symptoms of impending or developed cavernous sinus thrombosis includes:

- Worsening headache and facial pain
- Bilateral eye signs, proptosis of one or both eyes being an early sign
- Cranial neuropathies (III–VI, with nerve VI being the most common)
- Swinging pyrexia
- Symptoms not improving despite maximal medical therapy
- Worsening serological markers of infection

15. Answer C

Oral steroids are an effective acute intervention in patients with significant nasal obstruction due to polyposis. Additionally, by reducing polyp burden they also increase the nasal distribution of topical steroids. All the answers are known side effects of steroids; however, the most frequent of these in short courses are sleep and mood disturbance.

16. Answer B

Bevacizumab is a selective recombinant human antibody against VEGF, used for the treatment of metastatic colorectal, breast, renal cell and lung cancers. In the context of HHT, it can be used in a reduced dose intravenously to help those refractory cases that still require input despite maximal surgical and medical therapy.

17. Answer B

The posterior ethmoid and sphenoid sinuses drain into the sphenoethmoidal recess. The frontal, maxillary and anterior ethmoid sinuses drain into the hiatus semilunaris within the middle meatus.

18. Answer C

After exiting the sphenopalatine foramen, the sphenopalatine artery branches into the septal and posterolateral nasal branches, with the latter supplying the inferior and middle turbinate. The palatovaginal/pharyngeal artery is a branch of the internal maxillary artery.

19. Answer C

Sinonasal malignancies are associated with environmental risk factors. Patients with a history of woodworking or carpentry are more at risk of sinonasal adenocarcinoma. Historically, this was most prevalent in woodworkers in the furniture factories of High Wycombe. A background occupational history of nickel exposure increases the risk of primary sinonasal squamous cell carcinoma.

20. Answer D

In the UK, co-phenylcaine comes as a combination of lignocaine 5% and phenylephrine 0.5% in a standard 2.5 ml vial. Lidocaine 5% means 50 mg in 1 ml (a 1% solution is 10 mg in 1 ml). This therefore means that in 2.5 ml co-phenylcaine, there is 125 mg of lignocaine (50 mg in 1 ml x 2.5 ml).

21. Answer B

A keloid is an area of excess scar tissue that forms in response to a cutaneous trauma. Early keloids are composed of type III collagen and type I collagen predominates in more mature keloids. They differ from hypertrophic scars, which do not grow beyond the boundaries of the original injury.

Keloid scarring on the pinna can be challenging to manage, and selecting an appropriate treatment modality is essential for achieving the best cosmetic and functional outcome. Intralesional corticosteroid injections (e.g. triamcinolone) are considered a first-line option for reducing keloid size and symptoms on the pinna. It is an effective treatment to reduce both keloid size and symptoms including pain and itch. Excision with primary closure may be suitable for smaller keloids but carries a risk of recurrence if not combined with other modalities. Laser therapy can be used in combination with other treatments to improve the appearance of keloids but may not be as effective as corticosteroid injections alone. Silicone gel sheets can help prevent keloid recurrence after other treatments but are generally used as adjunct therapy. Radiation therapy may be used in refractory cases.

22. Answer B

When excising a squamous cell carcinoma (SCC) on the face, the appropriate excision margin typically falls within the range of 4–6 mm. The choice of margin width depends on various factors, including the size, location and clinical characteristics of the SCC, as well as the surgeon's judgement. This margin allows for the removal of the cancerous tissue along with a sufficient safety margin of healthy tissue to reduce the risk of tumour recurrence. SCCs on the face may require narrower margins compared to those on other parts of the body to preserve both function and cosmesis. A 4–6 mm margin strikes a balance between complete tumour removal and minimising cosmetic deformity while ensuring the best possible oncological outcome for the patient.

23. Answer D

A nasal mass with cervical lymphadenopathy is suggestive of malignancy. In this situation, primary site and staging scans are important, as is tissue sampling of the primary site (after imaging) and neck for nodal status.

Sinonasal malignancy in children is uncommon and should be managed within a paediatric MDT that includes ENT, oncology and radiology. Symptoms can often initially be subtle or non-specific, meaning that paediatric sinonasal malignancies are often diagnosed at a more advanced stage than in adults. Sarcomas are the most common sinonasal malignancy in children over the age of 10 years, of which rhabdomyosarcoma tumours are the most commonly diagnosed (with embryonal being the most common subtype). Malignant tumours of the sinonasal cavity in the paediatric population include:

- Rhabdomyosarcoma (or sarcoma tumours)
- Non-Hodgkin's lymphoma
- Olfactory neuroblastoma
- Nasopharyngeal carcinoma
- Primitive neuroectodermal tumours (PNET)

24. Answer E

A septal perforation commonly presents with nasal congestion, crusting, dry blood and often whistling due to turbulent airflow generated by eddy currents. This often improves as the perforation enlarges or crusting occludes the perforation. Cocaine use, digital trauma, tuberculosis and granulomatosis with polyangiitis (diagnosed with ANCA testing) are all known causes of a septal perforation but most commonly affects the cartilaginous nasal septum first and then extend posteriorly. Syphilis is the most likely condition in this scenario since it more frequently affects the posterior/bony septum and its treatment is easy with a low-risk antibiotic. Posterior perforations rarely cause a whistle and often go unnoticed by patients.

25. Answer B

An inverted papilloma (IP) is a benign sinonasal lesion associated with human papillomavirus. It is mostly associated with the HPV subtypes 16 or 18. Malignant transformation occurs in around 10% of cases. The mechanisms of malignant transformation are not well understood. IPs are mostly associated with the increased lifetime risk of squamous cell carcinoma, although cases of adenocarcinoma have been reported in the literature. Classically, IPs originate from the lateral nasal wall in the osteomeatal complex (OMC). Complete surgical excision remains the mainstay of management, with drilling of any hyperostotic site(s) and mucosal stripping undertaken to reduce the risk of recurrence.

26. Answer C

The carotid artery has been reported to protrude into the sphenoid sinus in 26.3% of patients. It is imperative that cross-sectional imaging is reviewed prior to performing endoscopic sinus surgery, particularly surgery of the sphenoid sinus.

Fadda, G.L., Petrelli, A., Urbanelli, A. et al. Risky anatomical variations of sphenoid sinus and surrounding structures in endoscopic sinus surgery. *Head Face Med* 18, 29 (2022).

27. Answer B

Hereditary haemorrhagic telangiectasia (HHT) or Osler-Weber-Rendu disease is an uncommon condition affecting roughly 1 in 5000 people in the UK and Europe. It has autosomal dominant inheritance and often presents with epistaxis and visible telangiectasia on the lips, face and hands and in the oral cavity. Central visceral organ arteriovenous malformations most often occur in the lungs, liver, GI tract and brain. Dysfunctional blood vessel maturation reduces effective vasoconstriction and hence increases the bleeding risk of telangiectasia. Diagnosis is based on the Curacao criteria, in which 2 criteria is probable and 3 is definite HHT:

- Epistaxis
- Telangiectasia on examination
- First-degree relative with the same condition
- Known central/visceral arteriovenous malformation

28. Answer C

Iatrogenic skull base injury associated with a CSF leak during routine endoscopic sinus surgery is rare: in the UK we commonly quote a figure of 1 in 5000 when consenting for routine endoscopic sinus surgery. Rates are understandably higher when related to complex procedures such as sinonasal tumour or skull base tumour resections, often anticipated to occur as part of the procedure in many cases. The anterior cranial fossa is the most common site of iatrogenic CSF leaks, and in particular the lateral lamella of the cribriform plate, which is the weakest portion of the skull base. This may be due to a breach as a result of powered instrumentation use, or aggressive manipulation of the middle turbinate intra-operatively.

29. Answer E

Reviewing the CT scan performed for sinus disease is crucial prior to considering endoscopic sinus surgery.

The Lund-Mackay staging system was developed in the UK and is used internationally to quantify sinus disease severity on CT scanning.

The scoring system assesses and scores the frontal, anterior ethmoid, posterior ethmoid, maxillary and sphenoid sinuses in addition to the osteomeatal complexes (OMC). It is undertaken for each sinus/side and is as follows:

- 0 is given for no opacification
- 1 is given for partial opacification
- 2 is given for complete opacification of each sinus
- 2 is given for blockage of the OMC
- Maximum score = 24

The correlation between Lund-Mackay scores and clinical severity is uncertain. However, higher scores may be associated with need for more extensive surgery. The Lund-Mackay staging system should be used in conjunction with the history, clinical examination and response to initial treatment, and it alone should not be used to determine surgical candidacy.

30. Answer C

Invasive fungal sinusitis (IFS), or mucormycosis, can be a life-threatening condition. It is more likely to occur in those who are immunocompromised such as patients with haematological malignancy, transplant patients on immunosuppression and diabetic patients (particularly those with poor control).

IFS is associated with reduced survival in patients with haematological malignancies, particularly when they are neutropenic with a count of less than 1.0×10^9/L. Neutropenia is a risk factor for poor outcome in other conditions, such as in sepsis. In these patients, ensuring their underlying pathology is managed is paramount, isolating them and starting IV antifungal treatment, such as Amphotericin-B, and granulocyte colony stimulating factor (G-CSF) can improve survival outcomes. IFS is considered a surgical emergency in situations of feasible debridement of dead/diseased tissue. When the disease has spread into the orbital cavity or intracranial cavity, debridement becomes less helpful and has a grimmer prognosis. Evidence of this can be seen via exam (in this case diplopia) or on imaging. IFS often presents with evidence of mucosal necrosis on MRI imaging (T2 dropout or lack of enhancement with contrast on T1). This alone is not a prognosticator, since surgical debridement may be feasible with an adjunctive antifungal therapy if the spread of the infection has not extended into the orbit or cranial cavity.

31. Answer D

Using the midpoint of the anterior lacrimal crest as a reference point, the anatomical relationships are as follows: anterior ethmoidal foramen (24 mm posterior), posterior ethmoidal foramen (36 mm posterior), optic foramen (42 mm posterior). An alternative way of thinking about these relationships is to remember that the anterior ethmoidal foramen is 24 mm from the anterior lacrimal crest, the posterior ethmoidal foramen is 12 mm from the anterior ethmoidal foramen, and the optic nerve is 6 mm away from the posterior ethmoidal foramen.

32. Answer D

The width-to-length ratio of a flap is crucial for ensuring its vascularity. For facial flaps, a ratio of 1:4 is generally recommended, while in the neck this is typically 1:2.

Several reasons justify a longer flap in the face compared to other body parts. The face has a rich vascular supply, with a dense network of anastomoses. This allows for the design of longer flaps with a narrow base without compromising blood supply. The face is also aesthetically sensitive. A longer flap allows for the redistribution of tension over a larger area, allowing the surgical site to align with the relaxed skin tension lines. This can result in a better cosmetic outcome with less visible scars.

33. Answer B

The primary treatment modality for squamous cell carcinomas (SCC) of the nose is surgical excision. Secondary intention or primary closure can be used to reconstruct narrow nasal skin defects. Larger defects are reconstructed with skin grafts or local flaps. Tip defects that are less than 1.5 cm in size and over 5 mm from the alar rim can be reconstructed with bilobed flaps, and cartilage grafts can be used to prevent alar notching as required. Smaller defects under 1 cm can be repaired using full thickness skin grafts, although skin colour mismatch should be considered. The paramedian forehead flap is the preferred choice in large, full thickness defects or those containing more than one nasal subunit. The paramedian forehead flap is staged over two or three sessions. It is an interpolated, axial-based flap pedicled on the supratrochlear artery.

If margins are reported as positive after the first stage, it is critical to re-excise to ensure complete removal of the malignancy. While the presence of a paramedian forehead flap complicates the scenario, ensuring oncological safety is the primary concern. Adjuvant treatments like radiotherapy might be considered in some cases of SCC, especially high-risk ones, but it is not the primary step after receiving a report of positive margins. Observation would not be appropriate given the known positive margins. Proceeding with flap surgery without addressing the positive margins could lead to recurrence. Sentinel lymph node biopsy is more common for melanomas and is not appropriate in this case.

34. Answer C

This is a very common question which can be asked in the FRCS (ORL-HNS) examination in both sections one and two. It is relevant for emergency, paediatric and rhinology cases. Chandler's classification is a method for describing severity of periorbital cellulitis and thus relevance for medical/surgical intervention. The Chandler classification (orbital complication of sinusitis) includes:

- Grade I: Inflammatory oedema (pre-septal cellulitis); normal visual acuity and extraocular movement
- Grade II: Orbital cellulitis with diffuse orbital oedema; no discrete abscess
- Grade III: Subperiosteal abscess of the lamina papyracea with downward and lateral globe displacement
- Grade IV: Orbital abscess with chemosis, ophthalmoplegia, and decreased visual acuity
- Grade V: Cavernous sinus thrombosis with progressive bilateral chemosis, ophthalmoplegia, retinal engorgement, and loss of visual acuity, along with possible meningeal signs and high fever

35. Answer C

Inverted papilloma is associated with HPV infection, specifically of the 6, 11, 16 and 18 serotypes. Serotypes 16 and 18 have been associated with a higher risk of malignancy. Malignancy should be considered when there is a rapid increase in tumour size, bleeding or invasion of adjacent structures. There is currently no consensus about the role of HPV infection in malignant transformation.

36. Answer B

Inflammatory nasal disease is the most common cause of changes in the sense of smell in the UK, and hence the most likely cause of hyposmia in this scenario. Olfactory disorders can be classified as conductive, whereby pathology blocks inspired odorants from reaching the olfactory cleft (e.g. rhinosinusitis or septal deviation), or sensorineural, caused by dysfunction of the olfactory receptor neurons or their central projections (e.g. trauma, viral infection, neurodegenerative disease).

37. Answer C

CT and MRI scans can help determine the tumour origin radiologically. CT scans are particularly helpful because they can assess for the hyperostotic area (or the stalk) of the inverted papilloma, as a likely indicator of the site of origin. Inverted papilloma most frequently arise from the lateral nasal wall, and often obstruct the middle meatus causing sinusitis symptoms, but since there is hyperostosis in the maxillary sinus, that is the most suspicious site in this case.

Inverted papilloma is the second most common benign tumour of the sinonasal tract after osteoma. Endoscopy usually shows a pale, polypoid lesion with a papillary appearance that protrudes from the middle meatus. The maxillary sinus is the most commonly affected sinus, but on occasion, the lesion extensively involves more than one sinus, making it difficult to assess for the exact site of origin. Opacification or fluid levels as signs of sinus infection do not necessarily indicate a site of origin.

38. Answer E

The clinical photograph shows a septal perforation. Initial therapy with nasal douching and rotational antibiotic creams or emollients can help improve symptoms dramatically, especially in the case of suspected prior recreational drug use. A haematological work-up to rule out vasculitis as well as urinalysis for cocaine metabolites in clinic are essential. A septal button or endoscopic repair with mucosal flaps (anterior ethmoidal or greater palatine artery based) may be considered for ongoing symptomatic perforations. Whilst failure rates were traditionally high, the advent of pedicled flaps has resulted in improved success, with some quoting 80% or greater closure rates for perforations up to 2 cm.

39. Answer A

Embolisation by interventional radiology can be helpful for patients that are not fit for formal surgical intervention due to other comorbidities and do not respond to standard medical treatment and nasal packing. The anterior ethmoidal artery is a terminal branch of the ophthalmic artery, which arises from the internal carotid artery, and is therefore not safe to routinely embolise due to the risk of blindness or a CVA. Branches of the external carotid system are considered safer to embolise.

40. Answer D

Based on the history, clinical findings and normal allergy testing, it is most likely that this patient is suffering with vasomotor rhinitis. Vasomotor rhinitis can quite effectively be treated with ipratropium bromide (such as Rinatec in the UK), which acts by blocking muscarinic acetylcholine receptors.

41. Answer C

The appropriate excision margin for a melanoma with a depth of 1–2 mm located on the face is 1 to 2 cm. This takes into account the thickness of the melanoma and recommends a margin that balances complete tumour removal with minimising excessive tissue excision.
Recommended margins:

- In situ melanoma = 5 mm margin (all removed)
- Melanoma less than 1 mm thick = 1 cm margin
- Melanoma 1 to 2 mm thick = 1 to 2 cm margin

- Melanoma 2 to 4 mm thick = 2 to 3 cm margin
- Melanoma greater than 4 mm thick = 3 cm margin

42. Answer C

A Z-plasty is a technique used to reorient and lengthen a scar. The angles of the Z-plasty determine the amount of lengthening possible as follows:

30 degrees: 25%

45 degrees: 50%

60 degrees: 75%

90 degrees: 125%

43. Answer E

The combination of an intranasal steroid and intranasal antihistamine has been shown to be superior to all other combinations of therapy. This combination reduces individual symptoms including nasal congestion, nasal irritation, rhinorrhoea and sneezing.

44. Answer D

Samter's triad (also known as AERD) is defined by three clinical features: asthma, sinus disease and recurrent nasal polyps, with sensitivity to aspirin and non-steroidal anti-inflammatory drugs (NSAIDs). These patients are complex and best managed with an MDT approach including ENT, respiratory and immunology. Biological therapies including benralizumab (Fasenra), omalizumab (Xolair), mepolizumab (Nucala) and dupilumab (Dupixent) are indicated in the treatment of chronic rhinosinusitis with nasal polyps and may be used in patients with AERD both before and after sinus surgery. Dupixent is an IL-4 and IL-13 blocking monoclonal antibody and based on efficacy and safety is considered the best choice of biologic for CRS. On the other hand, aspirin desensitisation is most effective if administered after sinus surgery. However, while aspirin desensitisation reduces the growth and recurrence of sinonasal polyps, it does not cause regression of existing polyps. Currently there is no evidence as to whether biological therapies are superior to aspirin desensitisation for AERD, and selected AERD patients may be considered for both therapies. It should be noted that currently the NHS does not fund biologics for the treatment of CRS although individual requests for funding can be made for CRS and they are available for selected patients with asthma. Aspirin desensitisation is also not widely available meaning comprehensive sinus surgery is critical for symptom control.

45. Answer C

This patient clearly has allergic rhinitis. Intranasal steroids and nasal douching remain the mainstay of management in most patients. Systemic absorption from topical steroid therapy, particularly in fluticasone, is as low as 0.5%. As a result, these can be pre-scribed without any concerns regarding systemic side effects and the patient can be counselled accordingly.

46. Answer A

The findings are consistent with Trotter's triad, which is a presentation associated with malignant tumours invading the lateral wall of the nasopharynx. Ipsilateral hypoglos-sal nerve palsy, abducens nerve palsy and trigeminal neuralgia are associated with

Godtfredsen syndrome, which is associated with nasopharyngeal tumours and can be seen in clival chordomas, meningiomas and metastatic disease.

47. Answer A

The likely origin here is the anterior ethmoidal artery (AEA), so this would be best tackled with an external Lynch-Howarth approach. The AEA is a branch of the ophthalmic artery, the first branch of the internal carotid artery. As such this rules out embolisation and external carotid artery ligation as viable management strategies.

48. Answer A

The UPSIT is used to test the function of a patient's olfactory system but can also be used in the diagnosis of pathology such as Parkinson's disease and Alzheimer's disease. The test has a total of 40 questions, consisting of 4 x 10 page booklets using a scratch-and-sniff system. Hence one would expect to score 10 (25%) by chance alone. The score is compared to a database of 4000 normal individuals, with a score of <5 indicative of malingering.

49. Answer A

In 1901 René LeFort described three transverse lines of weakness through the midface skeleton based on his experiments subjecting cadaveric heads to blunt force trauma. LeFort fractures are classified into three major types based on the pattern of the fracture lines and their anatomical relationships:

- LeFort 1 fracture (transverse): The fracture line runs horizontally just above the level of the nasal floor, and it separates the tooth-bearing portion of the maxilla from the rest of the maxillary bone. Clinically, this is evident as mobility of the upper teeth without involving the orbital rim or zygomatic arch.
- LeFort 2 fracture (pyramidal): This fracture line extends from the nasal bridge at or below the nasofrontal suture through the superior orbital rim, downwards towards the anterior maxillary sinus and crossing the pterygomaxillary fissure. Clinically, there can be a palpable step-off or depression at the infraorbital rim (known as an infraorbital step). This is in addition to the symptoms of a LeFort 1 fracture.
- LeFort 3 fracture (transcranial or craniofacial dissociation): This fracture line passes through the nasal bridge between the nasofrontal suture and the frontozygomatic suture line, extends laterally through the frontozygomatic process and the zygomatic arch, and then through the base of the pterygoid plates. This results in separation of the facial skeleton from the cranial base. Clinically, patients may present with CSF rhinorrhoea due to the involvement of the cribriform plate, in addition to facial mobility at the level of the nasofrontal suture and zygomatic arch.

In the scenario described, with the isolated mobility of the upper teeth and no other described clinical findings, a LeFort 1 fracture is the most likely diagnosis.

50. Answer C

The Abbe flap, also known as the lip-switch flap, is a full-thickness flap used primarily for the reconstruction of central lip defects. The flap is usually harvested from the opposite lip (for instance, using the lower lip to reconstruct a defect in the upper lip or vice versa). This allows for reconstruction of lip defects with similar tissue contained in the opposite lip. After transferring the flap to the recipient site, it remains attached to its original blood supply. The donor flap is pedicled on the labial artery of the opposite lip from the defect.

The flap is typically divided from its original location approximately 21 days post-operatively. This duration allows adequate time for establishing blood flow from the recipient bed, ensuring flap survival upon division.

51. Answer E

Morphoeic BCC is a high-risk cancer, with indistinct margins, and as such should be referred to your local dermatology unit responsible for Mohs micrographic surgery to ensure adequate margins. Primary closure is no longer recommended by the British Association of Dermatologists (BAD) and should be delayed until confirmation of clearance. In the event Mohs is not a viable option, an extended margin of 13–15 mm is recommended, with delayed closure.

52. Answer B

Basal cell carcinoma (BCC) exhibits diverse clinical and histological subtypes, each with unique characteristics. Nodular BCC is one of the common subtypes of BCC. It typically presents as a nodular lesion with a central ulceration surrounded by raised, pearly and translucent edges.

Other BCC subtypes:

- Superficial BCC appears as a well-defined, erythematous, scaly patch or plaque, often mistaken for eczema or a fungal infection.
- Infiltrative BCC lacks well-defined borders and may have a more aggressive growth pattern, making it challenging to delineate its margins.
- Morpheaform (sclerosing) BCC presents as a flat, scar-like lesion, often with indistinct margins, and can infiltrate deep into surrounding tissues.
- Pigmented BCC may resemble a melanoma due to its pigmentation, but it lacks the classic features of melanoma and shows histological characteristics of BCC.

53. Answer E

Lentigo maligna is a distinct subtype of slow-growing melanoma that typically occurs in the head and neck region of the elderly. It typically presents as a brown macule or patch. Histologically, it is typified by in situ growth by proliferation of atypical melanocytes along the dermal-epidermal junction. Rapid growth and metastasis, radial growth and irregular borders with various colours are features more commonly associated with other melanoma subtypes, e.g. superficial spreading melanoma and nodular melanoma. Keratin pearls are considered a marker of well-differentiated squamous cell carcinoma.

54. Answer C

A combination of CT and T2-weighted MRI (with CISS/FIESTA sequence) can localise defects in up to 95% of cases (CT alone will localise defects in 85% cases). Intrathecal fluorescein is an invasive test and is usually reserved for cases in which cross-sectional imaging including CT-cisternography fail to localise defects. Acetazolamide is considered in patients who have radiological features consistent with idiopathic intracranial hypertension.

55. Answer C

Paranasal sinus development starts following the development of folds along the lateral nasal wall at weeks 9–10 of gestation. Whilst up to 5–6 initially form, only 4 persist through regression.

> First: Uncinate and agger nasi
>
> Second: Middle turbinate
>
> Third: Superior turbinate
>
> Fourth/Fifth: Supreme turbinate

56. Answer B

Important concepts in the management of facial paralysis (of any aetiology) include early corneal protection (first and foremost priority), timely neurodiagnostics and possible surgical intervention. The question asks for the best long-term plan, so although Option A would be performed initially, Option B is a better longer-term plan. The patient likely had significant injury to the facial nerve during the procedure as suggested by the loss of signal during resection of the tumour. Therefore, it is expected that her facial nerve recovery will take months to years and a gold eyelid weight will assist with corneal protection during the period of waiting for any durable facial nerve recovery.

57. Answer E

Wallerian degeneration propagates distally from the site of injury to the motor end plate and proximally to the closest node of Ranvier. During first 3 days after injury, electrodiagnostic testing will be normal. After 72 hours, the distal aspect of the injured nerve will have denervated the muscle and be quiescent.

58. Answer D

Four constant Messerklinger landmarks exist: the uncinate process, anterior wall of the ethmoid bulla, middle turbinate basal lamella and the face of the sphenoid. There are also three inconsistent landmarks: ethmoid bulla posterior wall, superior and supreme turbinate basal lamella.

59. Answer E

The frontal recess is bound anteriorly by the agger nasi, posteriorly by the face of the ethmoid bulla, medially by the middle turbinate and laterally by the medial orbit.

60. Answer D

Tonometry will aid with diagnosis and post-treatment evaluation but offers very little in the way of initial management. Whilst mannitol, acetazolamide and dexamethasone are medical interventions that are described within the literature, they are unlikely to sufficiently reduce the intraocular pressure and prevent loss of vision. Time is of the essence in this instance, and immediate decompression with a lateral canthotomy and cantholysis is recommended. Should the intraocular pressures remain elevated, an endoscopic medial orbital wall decompression is the next stage in management. Nasal packing is contraindicated since it could impair drainage and worsen symptoms.

61. Answer B

Whilst no high-level evidence exists for the management of complicated acute frontal sinusitis, the consensus points towards surgical intervention. Given the location of the empyema, attention should focus on the affected frontal sinus, and in an acute setting a frontal sinus trephine with an outpatient review for definitive management is a reasonable option. Endoscopic Draf 3/modified Lothrop is usually reserved for aspirin-exacerbated respiratory disease (AERD) or lateral frontal sinus pathology.

62. Answer A

The patient has a juvenile angiofibroma (JNA) which is thought to have a relationship with testosterone production since it only presents in peri-pubescent males. It usually originates in the nasopharynx and often tracts into the pterygopalatine fossa leading to a Holman-Miller sign on imaging (anterior displacement of posterior maxillary wall). With patient history/demographic and imaging, one can diagnose the tumour without biopsy.

The Vidian artery is a branch of the internal carotid artery that travels with the Vidian nerve in the Vidian or pterygoid canal and enters into the pterygopalatine fossa often anastomosing with the external carotid artery system. The remaining options are all branches coming from the internal maxillary artery and would have likely been embolised with the pre-operative angiogram.

63. Answer A

Based on imaging and history, the patient likely has a mucocele from an obstructed frontal sinus outflow tract after a trauma. On imaging, mucoceles are T2 hyper-intense and T1 hypo-intense, homogenous, well circumscribed with expansile and erosive properties. Best management of mucocoele is marsupialisation and surgical assurance that a drainage pathway will be patent with an adequate frontal sinusotomy in this case. There is a chance this is caused by a tumour in the frontal sinus and the ESS would be a chance to biopsy and help guide next management steps at a later date. If it is a mass, resection is not indicated until knowing the pathology. Cranialisation of the frontal sinus is an option but endoscopic resection to diagnose and possibly treat the pathology has less morbidity and can be pursued at a later date if endoscopic management is unsuccessful. Trephination is used for frontal sinus osteomyelitis and anterior table erosion with Pott's puffy tumours. This may drain the sinus but would not improve the frontal sinus drainage pathways after healing. Antibiotics and steroids will not treat a mucocele or mass and are not appropriate in treating the patient's symptoms.

64. Answer D

Beclomethasone absorption is reported as high as 44%. As a side note, Budesonide is the only topical treatment that can be used in pregnancy, though recommendations are to avoid steroid therapy unless absolutely necessary.

65. Answer C

The segments described are as follows: C1: cervical, C2: petrous, C3: lacerum, C4: cavernous, C5: clinoid, C6: ophthalmic and C7: communicating. The most commonly injured segment during an endoscopic hypophysectomy is C4.

66. Answer B

Specific classification systems can be asked about in the FRCS examination. Krouse 1: Lateral nasal wall, Krouse 2: Ethmoids and maxillary sinus, Krouse 3: Frontal and sphenoid sinus, Krouse 4: Beyond sinuses. There is no Krouse 5 classification.

67. Answer B

The layers of the epidermis (deep to superficial) are stratum basale, stratum spinosum, stratum granulosum, stratum lucidum, stratum corneum.

68. Answer B

The histological findings are consistent with that of a clival chordoma. This is a rare, slow-growing tumour arising from notochordal remnants. Three subtypes exist: sacrococcygeal (most common), spheno-occipital and vertebral body. Metastatic spread is rare, occurring in up to 14% of cases. Symptoms are due to mass effect on structures such as the brainstem, cranial nerves, spinal cord and nasopharynx. Within the head and neck, the clivus is the most common location, and can be associated with an abducens nerve palsy due to its posterior location to the clivus. On cross-sectional imaging, these are usually midline tumours, with central calcification (chondrosarcomas are found off the midline). Whilst 5-year survival is poor at 40%, the mainstay of management is surgical resection and adjuvant radiotherapy.

69. Answer D

When addressing tip rotation, one must understand the concept of Anderson's tripod theory. In order to rotate the nose, you must shorten the lateral crura, or lengthen the medial crura. For this reason, a lateral crural steal will aid with tip rotation, but medial crural reduction will not. A septal extension graft will not only serve to provide additional tip support due to the short septum, but will also aid rotation, as will a strut graft. An ansa graft is sited at the caudal aspect of the dorsal septum in order to provide a higher attachment point for the lower lateral cartilages, thus increasing rotation and projection.

70. Answer A

The scan findings are consistent with a frontal sinus osteoma. These are usually slow-growing tumours found in 3% of CT scans, and are commonly found within the frontal > ethmoid > maxillary > sphenoid sinuses. They are the most common benign neoplasm of the paranasal sinuses, with a male predominance, and presentation most commonly occurs within the fourth to fifth decades. They are often incidentally found on CT, unless there is sinus outflow obstruction, or compression of critical structures. Gardner syndrome is a polyposis syndrome, which can be associated with multiple osteomas.

71. Answer D

Melanoma has a propensity to spread to regional lymph nodes, typically in a sequential manner. The sentinel lymph node(s) are the first nodes in the drainage pathway from the primary melanoma site. Sentinel lymph node biopsy (SLNB) is an integral part of the management of melanoma and enables the identification of the first regional lymph node(s) at risk of metastasis. The risk of finding a positive sentinel node increases with the melanoma thickness, number of mitoses and ulceration. Sentinel node positive patients have a higher rate of recurrence and worse overall survival.

72. Answer D

Differentiating between basal cell carcinoma (BCC) and squamous cell carcinoma (SCC) relies on clinical examination features as well as histology. Pearly or translucent appearance is more commonly associated with basal cell carcinoma (BCC) rather than squamous cell carcinoma (SCC). In contrast, SCC may exhibit different clinical characteristics including rapid growth and ulceration and central crusting.

73. Answer D

Whilst reconstruction varies amongst clinicians, a small defect within the anterior cranial fossa is likely to be low-flow, and thus robust reconstruction with pedicled flaps is rarely required (unless a revision case or a large defect). A nasoseptal flap is also unlikely to reach the superior aspect of the frontal sinus, whereas a pericranial flap is associated with significant morbidity, and is usually reserved for large defects following craniofacial resection. If a defect is identified, it must be repaired intra-operatively due to the low likelihood of spontaneous resolution.

74. Answer D

Allergic fungal rhinosinusitis is characterised by a type 1 hypersensitivity reaction. The Bent and Kuhn diagnostic criteria consists of 5 major and 6 minor criteria. A diagnosis of allergic fungal rhinosinusitis requires all major criteria be met. The minor criteria support the diagnosis but are not required.

Major Criteria: Type 1 hypersensitivity, nasal polyposis, characteristic CT findings (centrally hyperdense material with a peripheral rim of hypodense mucosa), eosinophilic mucin without invasion, positive fungal stain.

Minor Criteria: Asthma, unilateral disease, bone erosion, fungal cultures, Charcot-Leyden crystals, serum eosinophilia.

75. Answer C

All of the answers, with the exception of depth of invasion (≥2 mm is considered high risk) are high-risk features, which also include the presence of a lesion within the H-Zone of the face.

76. Answer E

The clinical and radiological findings in this case are consistent with an aggressive skull base malignancy and the patient has features of Foster-Kennedy syndrome (anosmia associated with optic atrophy/papilloedema due to raised ICP). The mnemonic 'MR SLEEP' can be used to remember tumours showing small round blue cell morphology: mesenchymal chondrosarcoma, melanoma, rhabdomyosarcoma, sinonasal undifferentiated carcinoma (SNUC), squamous cell carcinoma (including NUT carcinoma), small cell osteosarcoma, lymphoma, esthesioneuroblastoma, Ewing sarcoma/primitive neuroectodermal tumour (PNET), plasmacytoma and pituitary adenoma.

77. Answer E

Anterior cranial fossa spontaneous CSF leaks are commonly seen in patients with IIH. A rise in intracranial CSF pressures is thought to lead to dehiscence of the skull base in areas of presumed bony weakness such as the cribriform plate and the lateral lamella of the cribriform plate. Many neurosurgeons advocate a contrast MRI to rule out venous sinus thrombosis, which can be seen in spontaneous leaks. Hypertension is not a risk factor for the development of CSF leaks.

78. Answer D

Chondrosarcomas classically present off the midline in the clival region and can be challenging to manage due to their anatomical location. The mainstay of treatment is surgery followed by proton therapy, due to a reduced level of complications to surrounding tissue in comparison to traditional photon therapy.

79. Answer B

These are challenging cases, complicated more so in this scenario by pregnancy. Histological tissue sampling is crucial for the management of such cases and until tissue diagnosis is confirmed one should make every attempt to preserve vision where possible. In a similar scenario, maximal endoscopic debulking allowed for visual preservation and the histology was consistent with rhabdomyosarcoma, which was treated with chemoradiotherapy. Management of the pregnancy would require termination if the fetus were not a viable age for survival.

80. Answer C

This question tests the anatomy of the cavernous sinus. Structures on the lateral wall of the cavernous sinus from superior to inferior are the oculomotor nerve, trochlear nerve and the ophthalmic and maxillary branches of the trigeminal nerve. Structures passing medially are the internal carotid artery and abducens nerve.

The Knosp grading is a common system used to classify cavernous sinus invasion by pituitary macroadenomas. It is crucial in terms of operative planning to signify the likelihood of recurrence/residual tumour. Three lines are drawn (medial tangent, intercarotid line and lateral tangent) between the supraclinoid and cavernous ICA on coronal MRI sequences, which permit grading. Grade 3 tumours extend lateral to the lateral tangent (grade 3A extend above the intracavernous carotid the into the superior cavernous sinus and 3B extend below the intracavernous carotid into the inferior cavernous sinus). Complete encasement is a grade 4 on the Knosp classification. In the scenario described, extension into the superior cavernous sinus would be most likely to affect the oculomotor and trochlear nerves.

81. Answer A

Symptoms and signs of heavy metal poisoning vary according to the metal type and the chronicity of the exposure. Toxicity can result from acute exposure to large amounts or repeated exposure to small quantities. Heavy metals generate reactive oxygen species and subsequently cause oxidative stress to cells.

Arsenic poisoning is associated with a variety of dermatological and systemic manifestations due in part to the allosteric inhibition of pyruvate dehydrogenase, that converts pyruvate into acetyl-coA and is hence crucial to cellular respiration. Chronic exposure typically results from drinking contaminated groundwater. The highest groundwater arsenic levels have been recorded in Brazil, Cambodia, Afghanistan, Australia and Bangladesh.

Arsenic exposure can lead to the development of basal cell carcinoma (BCCs) and squamous cell carcinoma in situ, often on the trunk, and can result in palmoplantar keratosis, a condition characterised by thickening and scaling of the skin on the palms and soles. Mees lines, also known as leukonychia striata, are horizontal white lines that appear across the nails. They are typical of arsenic, thallium and selenium poisoning and have been reported in patients undergoing chemotherapy. They represent temporary interruptions in nail growth.

82. Answer B

Basal cell carcinoma (BCC) is the most common type of skin cancer, and can present in various subtypes, each with distinct characteristics. BCCs can be considered high-risk (morpheaform, infiltrative or basosquamous types) and low-risk (nodular and superficial types) depending on their invasive behaviour and recurrence risk. Clinically, morpheaform BCC present as a smooth flesh-coloured plaque or scar with ill-defined borders. It may be difficult to diagnose given that it does not resemble the typical nodular or superficial BCCs.

Morpheaform BCC secrete collagenases (matrix metalloproteinases), which enable them to invade and move between embryonic fusion planes (EFP) in the skin and cause local tissue destruction. EFPs are regions of mesenchymal and ectodermal fusion of the primordial facial processes. It has been suggested that EFPs differ in connective tissue structure from that of the surrounding area and hence facilitate deeper tissue invasion.

83. Answer B

The lymphatic drainage of the external nose primarily drains to the submental (Level IA) and submandibular (Level IB) nodes. Of these, the Level IB (submandibular) nodes serve as the major drainage point.

84. Answer C

A shortened columella is often seen in unilateral cleft lip patients post repair and can have significant aesthetic implications. A V-Y advancement flap is the favoured method for lengthening the columella in such cases. A V incision is made at the base of the columella, and the tissue is advanced upward, eventually being sutured in a Y configuration. This technique lengthens the columella without the need to introduce extra tissue. Another method is the lateral crural steal, which lengthens the columella by repositioning the lower lateral cartilages.

85. Answer C

The rhinion represents the most depressed point along the nasal bridge at the intersection between the nasal bones and the upper lateral cartilages. The thinnest skin of the nasal dorsum is sited here. This is an important consideration in rhinoplasty and post trauma as any bony irregularities will be visible. The radix is the soft tissue over the nasion, the point at which the frontal and nasal bones meet. The lower third of the nose and the glabella (the area of skin between the eyebrows) have thicker skin with more sebaceous tissue.

86. Answer D

Of overall complications following facelift surgery, haematoma formation is the most common, with an incidence of approximately 2%. Risk factors for post-operative haematomas include male sex, hypertension, and use of anticoagulants. Approximately 90% of haematomas occur in the first 24 hours after facelift surgery. Small haematomas can cause contour irregularities and pigmentation changes. A significant haematoma, such as one measuring 4 cm in diameter, can compromise the blood supply to the overlying skin flap. This can lead to devascularisation, and eventually skin necrosis. Although temporising measures such as suture removal and bedside hae-matoma drainage have been described, immediate evacuation in theatre is recommended to identify bleeding sites to relieve the pressure and ensure the survival of the flap.

87. Answer D

Rhinophyma is a subtype of rosacea characterised by erythema, telangiectasias and skin thickening predominantly of the lower third of the nose, leading to a bulbous, nodular appearance. It is more common in men and typically presents in the sixth to seventh decade of life. The exact aetiology is unknown, but it is not related to alcohol consumption, contrary to popular belief. While several treatment modalities can address rhinophyma, dermabrasion is often preferred for the best cosmetic outcome. This procedure involves mechanically shaving down the skin to improve its contour and appearance. It can be very effective in reducing the bulk and achieving a smoother, more refined nasal contour. Other treatments like topical agents and oral antibiotics mainly address inflammation and may not significantly improve the cosmetic appearance.

88. Answer D

Nasoethmoidal fractures involve the central midface. These fractures can result from high-energy blunt trauma, such as a motor vehicle accident. Clinically, they often present with telecanthus, a widened and flattened nasal bridge with increased inter-canthal distance. This is because the medial canthal tendons may be disrupted or detached, leading to an increase in the distance between the eyes. Clear fluid from the nose can be indicative of a cerebrospinal fluid (CSF) leak, which can be associated with these fractures due to proximity to the cribriform plate.

89. Answer C

Upper blepharoplasty is designed to remove excess skin (and sometimes fat) from the upper eyelids. Dermatochalasis is a term used to describe redundant eyelid skin and is a typical sign of periocular aging. Eyelid ptosis can be quantified by the margin-reflex distance-1 (MRD-1), measured from the midpoint of the upper eyelid margin to the centre of the pupil. The normal range is 4–4.5 mm and under 2 mm is considered ptotic.

When performing this procedure, it is essential to avoid excising too much skin, which can result in an inability to close the eye completely (lagophthalmos) or other complications, including scleral show. Typically, a maximum of 8–10 mm can be safely excised. The exact amount varies depending on individual anatomy and the degree of skin redundancy.

90. Answer D

The lateral helical rim-mastoid distance is ideally 2–2.5 cm with an auriculocephalic angle of 25–35 degrees; larger values are consistent with prominauris. The vertical height of the ear should be approximately 6 cm with a width 55% of its length. Prominauris generally results from an underdeveloped antihelical fold or less commonly excess conchal cartilage.

The Mustardé technique involves the use of permanent mattress sutures placed through the cartilage to create or enhance the antihelical fold. This is one of the most common techniques utilised for correcting prominent ears. The Furnas technique is used to correct excessive conchal cartilage by using four permanent sutures to secure the conchal bowl to the mastoid periosteum or cartilage of the ear (concho-mastoid sutures). The Stenström technique uses scoring or shaving of the anterior surface of the cartilage to weaken it, facilitating its reshaping. The Converse technique is a combination of cartilage excision and suturing to reshape the antihelical fold and reduce the conchal prominence. In the Davis technique, the hypertrophic cartilage of the posterior conchal wall and bowl are excised (usually involving a small kidney bean wedge of excess cartilage).

91. Answer C

Pemphigus vulgaris (PV) is an autoimmune blistering disorder that results from autoantibodies that target the keratinocyte adhesion proteins, desmoglein 3 (and sometimes desmoglein 1). This results in loss of cellular desmosomes, and a loss of cell-cell adhesion (with a histopathological finding of acantholysis and intraepidermal blistering). A genetic predisposition to PV has been linked with human leukocyte antigen (HLA) class II alleles (e.g. DQB1*0503 and DRB1*0402). Some cases may be drug-induced (e.g. captopril and non-steroidal anti-inflammatories). The disease initially presents with oral ulcers (80% of cases) which may rupture leaving painful erosions. Cutaneous blisters appear in about 75% of patients after the oral ulcers and are flaccid and rupture easily. The Nikolsky sign describes exfoliation of the outermost layer of skin with minor pressure. It is present in Stevens-Johnson syndrome (SJS), staphylococcal scalded skin syndrome, pemphigus foliaceus and PV. It is useful to distinguish between PV (in which the sign is present) and bullous pemphigoid (in which it is not). Corticosteroids are the mainstay of treatment of PV, but second-line treatment involves other immunosuppressants or biologics.

Bullous pemphigoid typically results in tense blisters, whereas PV leads to flaccid ones, and typically spares the oral mucosa. Bullous pemphigoid is associated with antibodies against hemidesmosome components, which lead to subepidermal blistering. Bullous impetigo is caused by the exfoliative toxin A produced by *Staphylococcus aureus* and causes reddish blisters on the skin of the face and chest which then burst leaving a honey-coloured crust. SJS is a mucocutaneous drug hypersensitivity reaction characterised by erythematous skin eruptions that progress to blisters and erosions accompanied by systemic symptoms, including sepsis, pneumonia and multi-organ failure. Erythema multiforme appears as red patches that evolve into target lesions most typically on the hands; it often results after infections (e.g. mycobacterium, streptococci, salmonella) or drug exposure (e.g. penicillin, sulphonamides, aspirin).

Given the presentation of painful oral ulcers, soft blisters, extension of blisters with lateral pressure and histopathological findings, the most likely diagnosis for this patient is PV.

92. Answer C

The external nasal skin is supplied by ophthalmic (V1) and maxillary (V2) branches of the trigeminal nerve (CN V) nerve. The infratrochlear (V1) and supratrochlear (V1) nerves supply the radix and cranial part of the dorsum. The external nasal branch of the anterior ethmoid nerve (V1) innervates middle vault and nasal tip.

The infraorbital nerve (V2) supplies the lateral nose and lateral tip. The nasal branch from the anterior superior alveolar nerve (V2) supplies the columella. Given the location of the pain, the patient is likely suffering from external nasal nerve neuralgia. It has been reported that this may respond to local anaesthetic blockade, with administration of local anaesthetic into the external nasal nerve which is found 6–7 mm lateral to the nasal dorsum at the level of the keystone area (where the nasal bones meet the upper lateral cartilages, as well as the cartilaginous septum and bony septum).

93. Answer D

Basal cell carcinoma (BCC) is a common skin cancer, especially on the face. The goal of treatment is to achieve complete tumour removal whilst maintaining function and cosmesis. The recommended margin for excision of a BCC on the face typically varies based on the clinical and histological characteristics of the lesion.

A number of surgical and medical therapies may be used to treat BCCs. For low-risk lesions (defined as low risk of recurrence, e.g. small nodular or superficial BCCs), these include electrodesiccation and curettage or surgical excision, topical 5-fluorouracil (5-FU) or imiquimod and photodynamic therapy. Mohs surgery, which combines staged resection under local anaesthesia with frozen section evaluation, is indicated for high-risk lesions at increased risk of recurrence and in functional or cosmetically sensitive areas. These would include lesions larger than 2 cm and aggressive subtypes such as infiltrative, morpheaform or micronodular.

For this low-risk lesion the 4 mm margin provides an appropriate balance between ensuring complete removal of the tumour and preserving surrounding healthy tissue for better cosmetic results. It allows for a safety margin to account for any microscopic extensions of the tumour beyond the visible margins and has been reported to achieve >95% tumour clearance rate. High-risk lesions generally require wider margins (5–10 mm).

94. Answer C

The diagnostic work-up for a potential melanoma on the neck is a critical process to evaluate the lesion's characteristics and establish the need for further intervention. Dermoscopy is a non-invasive diagnostic tool that allows for detailed examination of the skin lesion's surface. It provides magnified views of the lesion and facilitates assessment of various features including pigmentation patterns, borders and the presence of specific structures like globules and dots. This is important to distinguish between benign and potentially malignant lesions, including melanoma. Direct excision of the lesion to obtain tissue samples for histopathological examination should be considered only after a thorough evaluation, including dermoscopy, has raised suspicion of melanoma. Punch biopsy of suspected melanoma is not recommended. Clinical observation without intervention is not recommended for a potential melanoma, since early detection and biopsy are crucial for timely management. Sentinel lymph node biopsy is a procedure used to assess the spread of melanoma to regional lymph nodes and is typically not part of the initial diagnostic work-up.

95. Answer D

Chondrodermatitis nodularis helicis (CNH) is a painful condition characterised by a tender nodule or small lump on the helix or antihelix. It is commonly associated with trauma that causes localised vasculitis. Biopsy should be undertaken to distinguish from other benign or malignant causes, which may mimic CNH. Relieving pressure on the area with packing or padding is the mainstay of treatment although occasionally other modalities may be used, for example cryotherapy, intralesional steroids or laser excision.

96. Answer A

Full thickness skin grafts include the epidermis and entire dermis (with hair follicles). These grafts are useful in nasal, auricular and eyelid defects. Advantages of these grafts include better colour/texture/thickness match, durability, decreased wound contraction vs split thickness skin graft (STSG). Disadvantages include a higher metabolic rate, longer revascularisation time, decreased uptake percent compared to STSG and donor site morbidity. Graft survival depends on adequate recipient blood supply and patient risk factors (smoking, vascular disease, history of radiation). Graft failure can occur secondary to haematoma (most common), seroma, infection, graft mobility and wound tension.

97. Answer D

A paramedian forehead flap (PMFF) one/two/three stage axial flap is used mostly for nasal defects. It is based on the supratrochlear artery (identified at the supraorbital rim 1.7–2.2 cm from midline) which runs superficial to the corrugator muscle (divided during elevation) and deep to the orbicularis oculi, and pierces the frontalis muscle 2 cm superior to the rim. While it was initially described as a 2-stage procedure, the addition of a third intermediate stage has been introduced. Proponents of the 3-stage approach argue that the intermediate step improves flap perfusion, especially in smokers and patients with comorbidities that could compromise tissue healing (e.g. diabetes, rheumatologic diseases, vasculopathies). The 3-stage approach has also been purported to expand lining and structural support options and provide superior flap outcomes. There are also three varieties of the interpolated forehead flap: 1) paramedian: reputed to have increased dermal vascularity (despite similar viability) given centre position over pedicle with less desirable scar line than midline flap; 2) midline: offers a longer skin paddle with more favourable scar line. For the patient described, a midline forehead flap would reduce the need to go into the hair and hence bring hair down with flap; 3) single stage: limited to young, healthy patients without small vessel disease; requires de-epithelialisation and tunnelling under the glabella.

98. Answer C

Sellar defects and leaks are categorised as follows: Grade 0 (no visible leak on Valsalva), Grade 1 (mild leak, with no obvious diaphragmatic defect), Grade 2 (moderate leak with obvious diaphragmatic defect) and Grade 3 (high-flow leak with large diaphragmatic defect). The referenced paper provides an algorithmic approach for the repair of CSF leaks depending on leak grade.

Park JH, Choi JH, Kim YI, Kim SW, Hong YK. Modified Graded Repair of Cerebrospinal Fluid Leaks in Endoscopic Endonasal Transsphenoidal Surgery. *J Korean Neurosurg Soc.* 2015 Jul;58(1):36–42.

99. Answer B

Pitanguy and Ramos described a line starting from a point 0.5 cm below the tragus that extended in the direction of the brow, passing 1.5 cm above the lateral extension of the eyebrow. With this approximation, the nerve lies 2–3 cm from the lateral orbital rim at the level of the lateral canthus (Figure 4.6). Note the frontal branch is on the deep surface of the temporoparietal fascia when above the zygomatic arch. At the level of the arch, the nerve is relatively deep and adjacent to the periosteum.

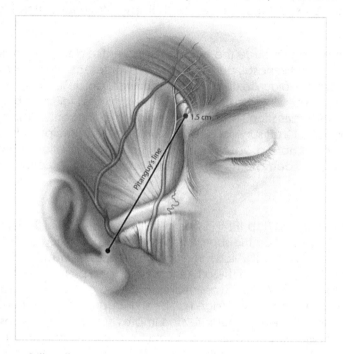

Figure 4.6 Pitanguy's line diagram.

Photo: https://plasticsurgerykey.com/4-frontal-branch-of-the-facial-nerve/

100. Answer B

The relevant and main parasympathetic neurotransmitter within the nose, which causes blood vessel vasodilatation, is acetylcholine. Over-the-counter nasal medications such as Xylometazoline cause vasoconstriction locally within the nose via adrenergic stimulation. This vasoconstriction leads to a reduction in soft tissue swelling and/or oedema, and as a result, improved nasal flow.

CHAPTER 5: EVIDENCE-BASED MEDICINE, STATISTICS AND MISCELLANEOUS

1. **A study into the effectiveness of a novel intratympanic drug for the treatment of sudden sensorineural hearing loss reports that the difference in hearing outcomes between the novel drug-treated group and the standard-of-care treatment group was statistically significant (p-value = 0.002). Which of the following statements is correct?**

   A   A p-value <0.05 means the difference is clinically meaningful

   B   The higher the p-value the more clinically meaningful the result

   C   The threshold for statistical significance is always p<0.05

   D   A p-value of 0.002 means that the result has a 99.8% chance of being true

   E   A p-value of 0.002 means the difference between the groups would have a 0.2% chance of occurring by chance

2. **A research study compared the olfactory dysfunction in men and women with COVID-19. At 6 months, the odds ratio of olfactory dysfunction in women compared to men was 3.1 (95% CI 1.2 to 9.4, p-value = 0.01). Which statement is correct?**

   A   Men experienced more olfactory dysfunction than women 6 months after COVID-19 infection

   B   Women experienced approximately three times the severity of olfactory dysfunction compared to men 6 months after COVID-19 infection

   C   The odds ratio of olfactory dysfunction in women is calculated by dividing the number of women with olfactory dysfunction by the number of men with olfactory dysfunction

   D   The odds ratio indicates that more women than men experienced olfactory dysfunction 6 months after COVID-19 infection

   E   A lower p-value means a more clinically significant difference in olfactory dysfunction

3. **You are wanting to investigate whether the choice of intranasal steroid affects the symptom control of chronic rhinosinusitis. You decide this is best approached by a randomised controlled trial (RCT). Which of the following statements is correct?**

   A   RCTs are better suited for retrospective analysis

   B   RCTs are particularly suited for the evaluation of rare outcomes such as the development of glaucoma with intranasal steroid usage

   C   Randomisation by online randomisation software can minimise the effect of confounding factors

   D   Using the first letter of the patient's name as a method of randomising patients would remove the chance of allocation bias

   E   An RCT design for this study is appropriate since RCTs require shorter follow-up periods

DOI: 10.1201/9781003455059-5

4. In a meta-analysis conducted to evaluate the efficacy of a tonsillectomy for treating recurrent tonsillitis, the researchers include studies with varying surgical techniques. Which statistical method is commonly used in meta-analysis to address this heterogeneity and provide a pooled estimate of treatment effect?
   A Sensitivity analysis
   B Funnel plot analysis
   C Fixed-effects model
   D Random-effects model
   E Stratified analysis

5. You are explaining the use of vestibular evoked myogenic potentials (VEMPs) in the investigation of superior semicircular canal dehiscence (SSCD) to a medical student. You explain that the test at your centre has a sensitivity of 85%. The medical student asked what this means. What is another way to explain this?
   A 85% of those with a positive test have SSCD
   B The test correctly identifies 85% of patients without SSCD
   C The test has a 15% probability to return a false positive result
   D 85% of those with SSCD will have a positive test result
   E The test is not reliable for diagnosing SSCD

6. You are designing a randomised controlled trial to assess the apnoea-hypopnea index (AHI) after cold steel and coblation tonsillectomy in children diagnosed with obstructive sleep apnoea. A sample size of 100 was calculated based on an 80% power to detect a 3-point difference in AHI. You were able to recruit 90 patients to the trial and you report that AHI was significantly lower in the coblation group (p-value = 0.04). Which of these statements is correct?
   A It is likely that there is a clinically meaningful difference in the AHI between the groups

B The power to detect a difference of 3 points was lower than 80%
C The trial was adequately powered to reject the null hypothesis
D The difference in AHI between the 2 groups is significantly larger than 3 points
E The trial should have been stopped if the number of recruited patients was less than 100

7. In a population-based study investigating the prevalence of laryngeal cancer among individuals who smoke and those who do not, what type of epidemiological study design is most suitable for assessing the association between smoking and laryngeal cancer risk?
   A Case-control study
   B Cross-sectional study
   C Cohort study
   D Randomised controlled trial
   E Ecological study

8. For which of the following situations would an independent sample t-test be appropriate?
   A Comparing patient body weight between those with and without tonsillitis
   B Comparing pain on a Likert scale before and after tonsillectomy
   C Comparing patient satisfaction before and after tonsillectomy for recurrent tonsillitis
   D Comparing the proportion of patients with recurrent sore throats in those who have had or have not had tonsillectomy
   E Comparing patient systolic blood pressure before and after tonsillectomy

9. You are analysing the results of your personal series of thyroidectomies. You find that the Pearson correlation between patient satisfaction and

length of stay is -0.7 (p = 0.01). Which of the following is correct?

A Longer patient stays were associated with greater patient satisfaction

B A correlation coefficient of -0.7 indicates a strong statistical significance

C There is a strong negative correlation between the length of stay and patient satisfaction

D There is a weak correlation between the length of stay and patient satisfaction

E A p-value of 0.05 would suggest a more statistically significant result than a p-value of 0.01

10. A journal article reports the result of a randomised controlled trial comparing vocal cord injection with a new bio-material to a placebo. They report the difference in voice outcome between the intervention and control group as measured on a 0–10 cm visual analogue scale (VAS) was 1.2 cm (95% CI -1.2 cm to 3.6 cm). Which of these statements is correct?

A 95% of the group treated with the new material had voice improvement of between -1.2 cm and 3.6 cm

B 5% of the control group had voice improvement of between -1.2 cm and 3.6 cm

C The improvement in voice outcomes of the new material could have been due to chance

D A VAS is an inappropriate tool for use with this type of data

E Estimating 99% confidence intervals would give a more accurate estimate

11. How much adrenaline is contained in 1 ml of 1:10,000 solution?

A 1 microgram
B 10 micrograms
C 100 micrograms
D 1000 micrograms
E 10000 micrograms

12. How much cocaine is in 10 ml of Moffett's solution containing 2 ml of 10% cocaine?

A 2 mg
B 20 mcg
C 200 mcg
D 20 mcg
E 200 mg

13. A 12-month-old baby weighing 10 kg undergoes microlaryngoscopy and bronchoscopy. During the procedure lidocaine 10% spray is used. If each spray delivers 10 mg of lidocaine what is the number of sprays that can be used?

A 1
B 2
C 3
D 4
E 5

14. What is the maximum safe dose of lidocaine that can be given to an 80 kg man?

A 240 mg
B 250 mg
C 320 mg
D 350 mg
E 560 mg

15. What is the maximum recommended safe dose of lidocaine with adrenaline?

A 5 mg/kg
B 6 mg/kg
C 7 mg/kg
D 8 mg/kg
E 9 mg/kg

16. A 45-year-old man with a prior history of myocardial infarction and atrial fibrillation undergoes tonsillectomy and you wish to administer a long-acting local anaesthetic for post-operative pain. Which of the following is the best option?

A Bupivacaine
B Levobupivacaine
C Lidocaine
D Cocaine
E Procaine

17. **You are performing a cricopharyngeal botulinum toxin injection for a patient with upper oesophageal dysfunction causing dysphagia. What is the mechanism of action of botulinum toxin?**
    A Inhibits the release of acetylcholine from pre-synaptic motor neurons
    B Inhibits the release of acetylcholine from post-synaptic motor neurons
    C Inhibits the reuptake of acetylcholine at the neuromuscular junction
    D Inhibits the release of GABA into the synaptic cleft
    E Stimulates the enzyme acetylcholinesterase

18. **You review a 65-year-old patient with profuse epistaxis. The patient is on warfarin for atrial fibrillation. Bloods reveal an INR (international normalised ratio) of 8. What is the best management option?**
    A Withhold warfarin
    B Withhold warfarin and administer oral vitamin K
    C Withhold warfarin and administer IV vitamin K
    D Withhold warfarin and administer prothrombin complex concentrate and IV vitamin K
    E Administer fresh frozen plasma

19. **You are asked to review a 30-year-old patient with tonsillitis who has received a stat dose of benzylpenicillin. The patient is hypotensive with lip and eyelid swelling. You suspect an anaphylactic reaction. What dose of adrenaline should be given?**
    A 0.5 ml of 1 in 1000 intramuscular (IM)
    B 0.5 ml of 1 in 1000 IM
    C 0.3 ml of 1 in 1000 IM
    D 0.3 ml of 1 in 1000 intravenous (IV)
    E 0.15 ml of 1 in 1000 IM

Answer A

As with any emergency, a rapid assessment of the airway, breathing and circulation (ABC) is essential. In cases of anaphylaxis, Option A should include removal of the allergen. According to the UK resuscitation guidelines the following doses should be administered:

Adrenaline (give intramuscular [IM] unless experienced with IV adrenaline). IM doses of 1:1000 adrenaline (repeat after 5 min if no better)

- Adult 500 micrograms IM (0.5 mL)
- Child more than 12 years: 500 micrograms IM (0.5 mL)
- Child 6–12 years: 300 micrograms IM (0.3 mL)
- Child less than 6 years: 150 micrograms IM (0.15 mL)

Adrenaline IV to be given only by experienced specialists: Adults 50 micrograms; Children 1 microgram/kg

20. **A 25-year-old patient with immune thrombocytopenic purpura (ITP) is due to undergo a parotidectomy for pleomorphic adenoma. At what threshold is a pre-procedural platelet transfusion indicated?**
    A $<5 \times 10^9$L
    B $<10 \times 10^9$
    C $<30 \times 10^9$
    D $<50 \times 10^9$
    E $<100 \times 10^9$

21. **Which of the following is true regarding a patient's living will/advance decision?**
    A Does not take precedence over decisions made in the patient's best interest by next of kin if legally binding
    B Does not need to be signed and witnessed if the patient is choosing to refuse life-sustaining treatment
    C Can be made by a patient without capacity
    D Can be used to request euthanasia
    E An advance decision is not the same as an advance statement

22. **With regard to xylometazoline which of the following is true?**
    A It is available in a 1% and 2% preparation
    B It is a beta adrenergic agonist
    C It is an alpha adrenergic agonist
    D It is most effective with prolonged use
    E It is a beta adrenergic antagonist

23. **In the UK, the Caldicott principles:**
    A Provide guidance on the use and protection of patient identifiable data
    B Relate to the safeguarding of children
    C Do not require all NHS organisations to have a Caldicott guardian
    D Relate to safeguarding of individuals at risk of being groomed or radicalised into terrorist activity, before a crime is committed
    E Do not apply to deceased patients

24. **A 40-year-old heavy goods vehicle driver has a history of acute episodes of sudden disabling vertigo associated with aural fullness and tinnitus. He continues to drive despite being advised to stop driving and inform the Driver and Vehicle Licensing Agency (DVLA). How should you proceed?**
    A Tell the patient's relatives to confiscate the patient's car keys
    B Inform the DVLA
    C Write a formal letter advising the patient not to drive again
    D Warn the patient that you will inform the DVLA if he has not done so by his next follow-up appointment
    E Inform the police

25. **A 50-year-old patient with profuse epistaxis requires blood transfusion. His blood type is A-. Which of the following blood types are compatible?**
    A A+, O-

B A-, AB-, O-
C A-, O-
D All blood types
E A-

26. **You see a patient who reports cold-like symptoms including nasal congestion, rhinorrhoea, sneezing and watery eyes over the past month. Radioallergosorbent (RAST) testing is positive for grass pollen. Which type of hypersensitivity reaction would most likely be evoked by grass pollen?**
    A Type I
    B Type II
    C Type III
    D Type IV
    E Type V

27. **You review a 36-year-old patient with an itchy erythematous rash on her hands. She reports this beginning since wearing rubber gloves. What type of hypersensitivity reaction is this an example of?**
    A Type I
    B Type II
    C Type III
    D Type IV
    E Type V

28. **A 24-year-old male undergoes a blood transfusion. He develops a morbilliform rash with itching. What type of hypersensitivity reaction is the patient experiencing?**
    A Type I
    B Type II
    C Type III
    D Type IV
    E Type V

29. **A patient with a history of chronic cocaine use is undergoing FESS. With regard to cocaine:**
    A Urinalysis for metabolites is positive for 2–3 days and may be positive for longer in chronic users

B Cocaine metabolites can typically be detected in blood or saliva for longer than in urine

C Patients with acute intoxication will be bradycardic and hypotensive

D Metabolic alkalosis is a complication of acute cocaine intoxication

E Troponin is not a useful test in patients with acute cocaine intoxication

30. **You are asked to review a 65-year-old female under investigation for right facial swelling, nasal obstruction and blood-stained rhinorrhoea. She becomes increasingly short of breath on the ward with increasing oxygen requirements (currently on 35% oxygen). The following is her arterial blood gas result, which is consistent with:**

paO$_2$: 7 kPa (11–13 kPa)

paCO$_2$: 3.5 kPa (4.7–6 kPa)

pH: 7.5 (7.35–7.45)

HCO$_3^-$: 23 (22–26 mEq/L)

BE: 0 (-2–+2)

A Respiratory acidosis

B Metabolic alkalosis

C Metabolic acidosis

D Metabolic alkalosis and type 1 respiratory failure

E Respiratory alkalosis and type 1 respiratory failure

ANSWERS

Evidence-Based Medicine, Statistics and Miscellaneous

1. **Answer E**

   A p-value is the probability of obtaining test results at least as extreme as those observed assuming that the null hypothesis is true. The null hypothesis (the alternative scenario to the study's hypothesis, e.g. that the drug improves hearing) is that there are no differences between the treatment groups. The p-value is the strength of the evidence against the null hypothesis but does not give an indication of effect size or clinical significance. P-values are most commonly considered 'statistically significant' when below 0.05 but can be varied depending on the study.

2. **Answer D**

   The odds ratio in this scenario is about comparing the frequency of olfactory dysfunction after COVID-19 infection in women compared to men. The odds represent the probability of having the event divided by the probability of not having it. They can be calculated by dividing the number of participants experiencing the event by the number not experiencing the event (i.e. the number of women with olfactory dysfunction divided by the number without). The odds ratio compares the odds of olfactory dysfunction in women compared to the odds in men. The odds ratio is above 1 and indicates that women participants report more frequent olfactory dysfunction at 6 months post infection.

   The p-value indicates the level of statistical significance and cannot be used to make inferences about clinical significance.

   An odds ratio is about the frequency of olfactory dysfunction and not the severity.

3. **Answer C**

   RCTs are considered the gold standard research method for assessing the effectiveness of interventions. RCTs involve random allocation of participants into treatment groups, ensuring that groups are comparable, and any observed differences in outcomes are due to the intervention being studied rather than confounding factors. This randomisation helps minimise bias and allows for stronger causal inferences. RCTs may or may not be suitable for evaluating rare outcomes since this is dependent on the sample size and duration of the study.

   Software- or online-based randomisation techniques are considered the best method of randomisation. The use of a patient name to randomise patients would be considered pseudo-randomisation and could be a source of allocation bias. RCTs are prospective studies and generally require longer follow-up periods to assess treatment effects adequately, not shorter ones.

4. **Answer D**

   In meta-analysis, when researchers include studies with varying interventions, effect measures or other sources of heterogeneity, a common statistical method used to provide a pooled estimate of treatment effect is the random-effects model which accounts for both within-study and between-study variation. It assumes that different studies may have different true treatment effects and incorporates this variability into the analysis. This model is suitable when there is heterogeneity among the studies.

This contrasts with the fixed-effects model that assumes that all included studies share a common treatment effect, and any observed variation is due to random error. It is appropriate when there is minimal heterogeneity among the studies.

A stratified analysis involves conducting separate analyses for subgroups of studies based on certain characteristics, such as study design, patient population or outcome measures. It can help explore sources of heterogeneity but may not provide a single pooled estimate.

Sensitivity analysis is used to assess the robustness of the meta-analysis results by testing the impact of different inclusion criteria or statistical methods on the overall findings. A repeat of the analysis is undertaken substituting alternative decisions for potentially arbitrary decisions taken in the included studies.

Funnel plot analysis is used to visually assess publication bias in meta-analysis. It can be used to assess whether there is asymmetry in the distribution of study results which may indicate publication bias.

5. **Answer D**

Sensitivity focuses on correctly identifying true positives (patients with the condition), while specificity addresses false positives (patients without the condition incorrectly identified as having it).

A sensitivity of 85% means the test would accurately identify 85 out of 100 people with SSCD. In other words, for 100 people with SSCD, we expect 85 to obtain a positive test result, and 15 a negative test result. The sensitivity does not tell us the probability of having SSCD for someone with a positive test result, which depends on the SSCD prevalence.

The sensitivity does not tell us about the proportion of false positive among those without SSCD, which depends on the specificity.

6. **Answer B**

The statistical power is the probability of detecting a significant difference if one exists. It is therefore the likelihood of correctly rejecting the null hypothesis when it is false. An 80% power means there is an 80% probability of detecting a difference if the true difference in AHI is indeed larger than 3 points.

The sample size is determined by several factors including the significance level, often denoted as α (alpha), that represents the probability of making a Type I error, which is incorrectly concluding that there is a significant effect when there is none. Commonly used levels of significance include $\alpha = 0.05$ (5%) and $\alpha = 0.01$ (1%). Other important factors include the effect size, variance of the outcome in the population and the statistical power of the study.

Given that only 90 patients were recruited based on a sample size calculation of 100 patients, this study had a power below 80% to detect a difference of 3 points on AHI.

7. **Answer A**

Case control studies are typically used to compare individuals with a specific condition (laryngeal cancer cases) to those without the condition (controls) and assess exposures retrospectively.

A cohort study is an alternative epidemiological study design for assessing the association between smoking and laryngeal cancer risk in a population-based study. Cohort studies follow a group of individuals over time, collecting data on exposures (e.g. smoking) and outcomes (e.g. laryngeal cancer). This design allows for the assessment of associations, the determination of temporal relationships and the calculation of relative risks. However, since laryngeal cancer is relatively rare, a large cohort of patients would be required, making this a less favourable design than a case control study.

Cross-sectional studies aim to provide data on an entire population at a single point in time, making them less suitable for assessing causality or tracking exposures and outcomes over time. Randomised controlled trials involve random allocation of participants to treatment groups and are more commonly used for interventions rather than epidemiological investigations of risk factors. It would also not be ethically possible to randomised participants to smoking or not. Ecological studies examine population-level data and are less suitable for assessing individual-level associations, such as the relationship between smoking and laryngeal cancer risk.

8. **Answer A**

Answer A compares a continuous variable between two independent groups (those with tonsillitis and those without) so an independent sample t-test is appropriate.

Answers B, C and E would require a paired sample t-test, since the before and after groups are the same patient group and are thus paired. Answer D requires a test of proportion such as chi-squared test.

9. **Answer C**

A Pearson correlation coefficient of -0.7 indicates a strong negative correlation between two variables, in this case, between length of stay and patient satisfaction. The correlation coefficient, r, can be between +1 and -1, with +1 indicating a perfect positive correlation and -1 a perfect negative correlation. The p-value of 0.01 suggests that this correlation is statistically significant, meaning it is unlikely to have occurred by chance. A p-value of 0.05 would suggest a less statistically significant result than a p-value of 0.01.

10. **Answer C**

A visual analogue scale (VAS) is a psychometric response scale and a well-accepted method by which to measure subjective experience such as pain or voice outcomes.

A 95% confidence interval (CI) is a range of values that likely contains the true value of a parameter with a 95% probability. A 99% CI would be more likely to contain the true estimate (99% likely) but would result in a wider (less precise) interval. Since the confidence interval here includes zero, we cannot rule out that the observed treatment effect (higher VAS in the patients treated with the new material) was only due to chance.

Reference: Naunheim MR, Dai JB, Rubinstein BJ, Goldberg L, Weinberg A, Courey MS. A visual analog scale for patient-reported voice outcomes: The VAS voice. *Laryngoscope Investig Otolaryngol.* 2019 Dec 17;5(1):90–95. doi: 10.1002/lio2.333.

11. **Answer C**

In a 1:10,000 adrenaline ampoule there is 1 part adrenaline to 10,000 parts solution. To work out how many micrograms (mcg) of adrenaline are present:

    1 mcg = 0.000001 grams (g) or 0.001 milligrams (mg)

    1:10,000 solution adrenaline

        = 1 g adrenaline in 10,000 ml solution

        = 1000 mg per 10,000 ml

$$= 1 \text{ mg per 10 ml}$$
$$= 0.1 \text{ mg per 1 ml}$$
$$= 100 \text{ mcg per 1 ml}$$

12. Answer E

10% solution of cocaine

$$= 10 \text{ g in 100 ml}$$
$$= 10{,}000 \text{ mg per 100 ml}$$
$$= 100 \text{ mg per 1 ml}$$
$$= 200 \text{ mg per 2 ml}$$

13. Answer C

To determine the number of sprays, we can calculate the safe dose of lidocaine based on the baby's weight. A dose of 3 mg/kg lidocaine is considered appropriate for paediatric airway topicalisation.

Safe dose of lidocaine = 3 mg/kg x weight (in kg)

Safe dose of lidocaine = 3 mg/kg x 10 kg

Safe dose of lidocaine = 30 mg

Since each spray delivers 10 mg of lidocaine, we can divide the maximum safe dose by the amount of lidocaine delivered per spray:

Number of sprays = 30 mg/10 mg per spray

Number of sprays = 3

14. Answer A

Safe dose of lidocaine = 3 mg/kg x weight (in kg)

Safe dose of lidocaine = 3 mg/kg x 80 kg

Safe dose of lidocaine = 240 mg

15. Answer C

Table 5.1

Anaesthetic	Maximum safe dose
Bupivacaine	2 mg/kg
Bupivacaine with adrenaline	2 mg/kg
Lidocaine	3 mg/kg
Lidocaine with adrenaline	7 mg/kg

16. Answer B

Levobupivacaine is a long-acting local anaesthetic. It is an isomer of bupivacaine. Whilst the anaesthetic and analgesic properties are similar to bupivacaine it is associated with less cardiotoxicity.

17. Answer A

Botulinum toxin is a highly potent neurotoxin produced by the Gram-positive bacteria *Clostridium botulinum*. It can be used for therapeutic and cosmetic purposes. It acts by causing inhibition of the release of acetylcholine from presynaptic motor neurons.

Specifically, it cleaves SNARE proteins, required for neurotransmitter exocytosis, resulting in flaccid paralysis.

18. Answer D

Supratherapeutic INR and major bleeding secondary to warfarin therapy requires complete anticoagulation reversal immediately. Warfarin is a vitamin K dependant clotting factor (II, VII, IX and X) inhibitor. The goal of reversal is to increase the available amount of vitamin K dependent clotting factors resulting in a decrease in INR. In ascending order of potency reversal can be achieved by withholding warfarin and administering oral or IV vitamin K and prothrombin complex concentrate (PCC) which contains vitamin K dependant clotting factors. Of note, PCC can cause thrombosis and disseminated intravascular coagulation given that patients receiving warfarin likely have an underlying hypercoagulable state. If PCC is not available or is contraindicated, fresh frozen plasma (FFP) can be administered; however, it is not the optimal agent given that PCC is more effective and rapid in action, is associated with a shorter preparation time since it does not need to be thawed and has a greater increase in clotting factors, does not require blood type matching, is infused at a faster rate than FFP with less volume and is associated with fewer complications due to fluid overload.

19. Answer A

As with any emergency, a rapid assessment of the airway, breathing and circulation (ABC) is essential. In cases of anaphylaxis, Option A should include removal of the allergen. According to the UK resuscitation guidelines the following doses should be administered:

Adrenaline (give intramuscular [IM] unless experienced with IV adrenaline) IM doses of 1:1000 adrenaline (repeat after 5 min if no better).

- Adult 500 micrograms IM (0.5 mL)
- Child more than 12 years: 500 micrograms IM (0.5 mL)
- Child 6–12 years: 300 micrograms IM (0.3 mL)
- Child less than 6 years: 150 micrograms IM (0.15 mL)

Adrenaline IV to be given only by experienced specialists: Adults 50 micrograms; Children 1 microgram/kg

20. Answer D

ITP is an autoimmune disease characterised by a low platelet count and purpura in the absence of an identifiable cause. In approximately 60% of cases, antibodies against platelets can be found. According to the British Society for Haematology a platelet threshold of 50 x 10^9 is recommended prior to major surgery.

21. Answer E

An advanced decision to refuse treatment (living will) is a legal document outlining a patient's healthcare preferences in the event they lose capacity to make these decisions. It allows a person to choose which medical treatments they wish to refuse including life-sustaining treatments such as CPR and ventilation. It is not the same as an advance statement which is a more general statement regarding one's preferences, wishes, beliefs and values regarding future care, e.g. preference to be cared for at home vs in hospice. For an advance decision to be legally binding it must comply with the Mental Capacity Act, be valid (patient aged 18 or older, clearly stating which treatments one wishes to refuse under which circumstances, signed by the patient and a witness if refusing life-sustaining treatment) and be applicable to the situation. If legally binding, it cannot be overruled by next of kin.

22. Answer C

Xylometazoline is a sympathomimetic and acts directly as an alpha adrenergic agonist. It is used for the temporary relief of nasal congestion. It is available as a 0.05% preparation for children aged 6–11 and 0.1% for adults. With prolonged use, rebound congestion (rhinitis medicamentosa) results and subsequently a temporary increase in nasal congestion symptoms.

23. Answer A

The Caldicott principles were first introduced in 1997 and have since been expanded. They are a set of good practice guidelines for using and protecting patient identifiable data. At an organisational level, Caldicott guardians support the upholding of the principles.

- Principle 1: Justify the purpose(s) for using confidential information.
- Principle 2: Use confidential information only when it is necessary.
- Principle 3: Use the minimum necessary confidential information.
- Principle 4: Access to confidential information should be on a strict need-to-know basis.
- Principle 5: Everyone with access to confidential information should be aware of their responsibilities.
- Principle 6: Comply with the law.
- Principle 7: The duty to share information for individual care is as important as the duty to protect patient confidentiality.
- Principle 8: Inform patients and services users about how their confidential information is used and what choice they have. There should be no surprises.

24. Answer B

The DVLA states that people who experience sudden, disabling or recurrent dizziness should stop driving and inform the DVLA. The driver is legally responsible for telling the DVLA. It is the doctor's duty to inform the patients to tell the DVLA. However, if an unfit patient continues to drive doctors may need to disclose this to DVLA without consent in the interest of the public.

25. Answer C

Red blood cells have cell surface antigens which can incite an immune response potentially resulting in transfusion reactions (see Table 5.2). Consideration of the ABO and RhD groups is very important to prevent incompatible blood transfusions.

Table 5.2

Blood type	Can donate to	Can receive from
A+	A+, AB+	A+, A-, O+, O-
A-	A-, A+, AB+, AB-	A-, O-

(Continued)

Table 5.2 (Continued)

Blood type	Can donate to	Can receive from
B+	B+, AB+	B+, B-, O+, O-
B-	B-, B+, AB+, AB-	B-, O-
AB+	AB+	All blood types
AB-	AB-, AB+	AB-, A-, B-, O-
O+	O+, A+, B+, AB+	O+, O-
O-	All blood types	O-

26. **Answer A**

Hypersensitivity reactions are inappropriate or exaggerated immunologic responses triggered by allergens or antigens. Type I hypersensitivity is an immediate and self-limiting reaction, mediated by the IgE antibody. Following sensitisation, repeat encounter with antigens results in IgE stimulating mast cells and basophils to release histamine, serotonin and other mediators. It results in allergy, anaphylaxis and atopic disease.

27. **Answer D**

Type IV hypersensitivity is also known as delayed hypersensitivity. It is mediated by T-cells. Contact dermatitis and the Mantoux test are examples of a type IV hypersensitivity reaction.

28. **Answer B**

Type II hypersensitivity is an IgG or IgM antibody-mediated cytotoxic reaction. Examples include transfusion reactions, Goodpasture's syndrome and haemolytic anaemia See Table 5.3.

Table 5.3

Hypersensitivity reaction type	Mediators	Timeframe	Examples
I (immediate)	IgE	Immediate	Hayfever, asthma, eczema, food allergies, anaphylaxis
II (Cytotoxic, antibody-dependent)	IgG, IgM	Hours to days	Autoimmune haemolytic anaemia, haemolytic disease of the newborn, Goodpasture's syndrome, acute transfusion reactions
III (Immune complex disease)	IgG, IgM, antigen aggregates, complement	Hours to days/weeks	Glomerulonephritis, rheumatoid arthritis, systemic lupus erythematosus
IV (Delayed hypersensitivity reaction – cell-mediated, antibody-independent)	T-cells, macrophages, monocytes	Delayed (24–72 hours)	Contact dermatitis, tuberculin skin test, chronic transplant rejection

29. **Answer A**

    Cocaine metabolites can usually be detected in saliva and blood for up to 48 hours and in urine for 72 hours. However, in chronic users, urinalysis may be positive for 2–3 weeks. Cocaine is a sympathomimetic, thereby causing tachycardia and hypertension in acute toxicity. It results in a metabolic acidosis. Myocardial infarction is a risk of intoxication and therefore troponin is a useful test.

30. **Answer E**

    Looking at the pH, the patient is alkalotic. $paCO_2$ is low contributing to alkalosis. HCO_3^- is normal as is the base excess (BE). Therefore, the metabolic system is not contributing to the alkalosis and there is no metabolic compensation. The patient is hypoxaemic with a paO_2 <8 kPa despite 35% oxygen consistent with type 1 respiratory failure.

Index

A

Abbe flap, 154
abnormal perchlorate discharge test, 87
absent cochlear nerve, 120
acetazolamide, 155
acoustic brainstem responses (ABR), 13, 25
acute facial palsy, 45
acute lymphoblastic leukaemia (ALL),
    125–126
acute myeloid leukaemia, 129
acute otitis media, 31, 114
acute vertigo, 11
adenoid cystic carcinoma, 60
adenoidectomy, 98
airway, breathing and circulation (ABC),
    177
airway endoscopy, 106
Alexander's law, 35
allergic fungal rhinosinusitis, 159
Alport syndrome, 112
alveolar rhabdomyosarcoma, 111
Annie nuclei, 79–80
anterior ethmoidal artery (AEA), 154
anterior lacrimal crest, 150
anterolateral thigh flap (ALT), 81
Apert syndrome, 103
apnoea-hypopnea index (AHI), 82, 168
Arnold's nerve, 22
arsenic exposure, 160
arsenic poisoning, 160
arteritic anterior ischemic optic neuropathy
    (AAION), 72
aspirin, 153
aspirinexacerbated respiratory disease
    (AERD), 157
atresiaplasty, 4
atypical mycobacterial lymphadenitis, 112
audiogram, 24, 34
auditory brainstem implant (ABI), 47
auditory brainstem response (ABR), 24
auditory nerve and brainstem evoked
    potentials (ABEP), 100, 120
auditory neuropathy spectrum disorder
    (ANSD), 38
auto-atticotomy cavity, 9
automated otoacoustic emissions (AOAE),
    6, 29
auto-myringostapedopexy, 29
autophony, 12
awake flexible laryngoscopy, 117

B

bacterial meningitis, 5
basal cell carcinoma (BCC), 133, 137, 155,
    158, 161
beclomethasone absorption, 157
Bell's palsy, 45, 53
bendroflumethiazide, 11
benign paroxysmal positional vertigo
    (BPPV), 39
Benjamin Inglis classification, 101
benzylpenicillin, 170
beta-2-transferrin, 133, 145
betahistine, 11
bevacizumab (avastin), 42–43, 126, 147
bicoronal osteoplastic flap, 55
bilateral acute otitis media, 33
Bilateral choanal atresia, 114
bilateral downsloping hearing loss, 5
bilateral lymphadenopathy, 67
bilateral nasal polyposis,
    112
bilateral sensorineural hearing loss, 4
bilateral symmetrical downsloping hearing
    loss, 6
Bill's bar, 44
biphasic stridor, 116
blilateral parotid swelling, 75
blind sac closure, 1, 7, 31
blistering rash, 65
bone-anchored hearing aid (BAHA),
    4–5, 26
botulinum toxin, 170, 176
botulinum toxin A, 81
Boyce's sign, 77
brain fog, 12, 20, 50
branchial arch system, 102–103
branchial system anomaly, 95
branch of the superior laryngeal nerve
    (EBSLN), 79–80
breast cancer, 17
Brown's sign, 31
bullous pemphigoid, 163

C

Caldicott principles, 171, 178
Candida albicans, 83
carotid artery, 149
cartilage tympanoplasty, 33
central nervous system (CNS), 109
cerebellopontine angle (CPA), 16, 17
    ependymomas, 44
    translabyrinthine approach, 42
cerebrospinal fluid (CSF), 16, 28, 42
    gusher, 47
    IIH, 143
    leak, 13, 46, 49, 125, 137
cervical VEMPs (cVEMPs), 50
Chandler classification, 151
CHARGE syndrome, 114
chemo-radiotherapy, 9
chemotherapy, 2, 4, 24
choanal atresia, 94
cholesteatoma, 8, 10, 12, 33, 35
chondrodermatitis nodularis helicis (CNH), 164–165
chondrosarcomas, 159–160
chronic mucosal otitis, 13
chronic nasal obstruction, 93
chronic obstructive pulmonary disease (COPD), 67
chronic rhinitis, 131
chronic rhinosinusltis, 132
chronic rhinosinusitis with nasal polyposis (CRSwP), 126
chronic rhinosinusitis without nasal polyps (CRSsNP), 143
chronic suppurative otitis media, 13
chyle leak, 85
ciloxan, 29
cisplatin, 24
Clostridium botulinum, 176
cocaine metabolites, 180
cochlear implantation, 2, 18
cochlear implant complications, 48
Collins syndrome, 14
compensatory tachycardia, 120
completely-in-canal (CIC), 27
compound muscle action potential (CMAP), 45
conductance regulator gene (CFTR), 112
congenital aural atresia, 26, 107
congenital midline craniofacial masses, 110
congenital piriform sinus fistula, 115
congenital stenosis, 117
congenital subglottic stenosis, 97
congenital tracheal stenosis (CTS), 100, 120

congenital tracheoesophageal fistula, 113
congenital vocal fold paralysis, 109
contact dermatitis, 38, 179
continuous positive airway pressure device (CPAP), 58
contralateral routing of sound (CROS), 27
co-phenylcaine, 147
coronal cranial sutures, 87
cortical evoked response audiometry (CERA), 24–25
cortical mastoidectomy, 88
corticosteroids, 109
Cottle manoeuvre, 123
Cotton-Myer classification, 92
Cotton-Myer grading scale, 110
COVID-19 infections, 130, 132, 167, 173
craniosynostosis, 103
C-reactive protein (CRP), 10, 18, 130
cystic fibrosis (CF), 112

D

dacryocystorhinostomy (DCR), 132
delayed-onset (rather than immediate) facial palsy, 23
dementia, 65
depth of invasion (DOI), 84
dexamethasone, 23
diffusion weighted MRI (dwMRI), 9, 21
DiGeorge syndrome, 104
digital modulation (DM) system, 29
dilatory Eustachian tube dysfunction, 31
diphtheria anti-toxin, 84
distortion product OAE (DPOAE), 25
Dix-Hallpike manoeuvre, 14
Dix-Hallpike test, 11
dizziness, 20
driver and vehicle licensing agency (DVLA), 171, 178
drooling, 108–109
dysphagia, 92
dysphonia, 54
dyspnoea, 91

E

EAC cholesteatoma, 40
ear itching, 5
electromyography (EMG), 45
    guided Botox injections, 21
electroneuronography (ENoG), 45, 49
embryonic fusion planes (EFP), 161
endotracheal tube (ETT), 97

enlarged vestibular aqueduct (EVA), 47, 48, 111
ependymomas, 44
epidermis, 158
epistaxis, 131
Epley manoeuvre, 36
Epstein-Barr virus (EBV), 54, 73
erythrocyte sedimentation rate (ESR), 54
European Laryngological Society classification, 71
Eustachian tube dysfunction (ETD), 21, 29, 98
Eustachian tube orifice, 31
examination under anaesthesia (EUA), 128
exostoses, 40
external auditory canal (EAC), 31
    air conduction (AC) sounds, 41
    bone conduction (BC) sounds, 41
    malignancy, 41

F

facial nerve dehiscence, 31
facial nerve palsy, 55, 59
facial palsy, 7
facial paralysis, 156
facial schwannoma, 45
familial adenomatous polyposis (FAP), 85
fine needle aspiration (FNA), 61
fistula test, 11
flexible endoscopic evaluation of swallowing (FEES), 107
flexible laryngoscopy, 97
flucloxacillin, 93
fluticasone, 109
follicular carcinoma, 79
frequency modulation (FM) system, 29
fresh frozen plasma (FFP), 177
Frey's syndrome, 81
Friedman staging system, 82
full thickness skin grafts, 165
functional endoscopic sinus surgery (FESS), 134, 137, 171
Furstenberg's sign, 94, 113
Fusobacterium necrophorum, 114

G

gadolinium enhancement, 76
Gallium scans, 34
Gardasil, 79
gastric ulcers, 10

gastroesophageal reflux disease (GORD), 103
gentisone HC, 29
giant cell arteritis (GCA), 72
glossopharyngeal nerve, 75, 77
glottic SCC, 69
Goldenhar syndrome (hemifacial microsomia), 49
Granular myringitis, 39
Griesinger's sign, 31

H

Haberman design, 118
haematoma formation, 161
Haemophilus influenzae, 37, 39
head and neck cancer, 58
head and neck lymphadenopathy, 60
hemithyroidectomy, 56, 61, 63
Hennebert's sign, 31, 111
hereditary haemorrhagic telangiectasia (HHT), 126, 149
Hitselberger's sign, 31
HIV, 66
Hodgkin's lymphoma, 108
holoprosencephaly (HPE), 103
HPV strain 16, 77
human papillomavirus (HPV), 59
hydrocephalus, 43
hypercalcaemia, 54
hyperkalaemia, 79
hypersensitivity, 179
hypertension, 4, 57, 65
hypopharyngeal SCC, 60, 63
hypothalamic-pituitary-adrenal (HPA), 109
Hyrtl's fissure (tympanomeningeal fissure), 13, 37

I

iatrogenic facial palsy, 30
iatrogenic skull, 149
idiopathic intracranial hypertension (IIH), 143
immune thrombocytopenic purpura (ITP), 170, 177
inducible laryngeal obstruction, *see* paradoxical vocal cord dysfunction
infantile subglottic haemangiomas, 107
infected osteoradionecrosis, 22
inferior turbinate hypertrophy, 109, 144
inflammatory markers, 19
inflammatory nasal disease, 151

intensity modulated radiation therapy (IMRT), 52, 69
internal auditory canal (IAC), 43, 47
internal auditory meatus (IAM), 17, 42, 44
internal jugular vein (IJV), 35
in-the-canal (ITC), 27
intracanalicular vestibular schwannoma, 5
intracranial infections, 87, 102
intratympanic steroids, 34
invasive fungal sinusitis (IFS), 150
inverted papilloma, 151, 152
inverted papilloma (IP), 148
invisible-in-canal (IIC), 27
ipsilateral cochlear implantation, 21
ipsilateral House-Brackmann grade IV facial palsy, 15, 17, 45
ipsilateral vestibulocochlear nerve, 21
IV chemotherapy, 2

J

Jacobson's nerve, 22
Jahrsdoerfer grading, 19, 49
Jahrsdoerfer grading scale, 108
Jehovah's Witness Liaison Committee (JWLC), 110, 111
Joll's triangle, 79–80
juvenile nasopharyngeal angiofibroma (JNA), 104, 157
juvenile-onset recurrent respiratory papillomatosis, 121

K

keloid, 147
keratoacanthoma (KA), 77
keratosis obturans, 40
Klebsiella rhinoscleromatis, 146

L

labyrinthectomy, 35
labyrinthine fistula, 8, 32
labyrinthitis, 35
laryngeal cancer, 2, 66
laryngeal cleft, 121
laryngeal injury, 53
laryngeal keels, 117
laryngeal reinnervation, 107
laryngomalacia, 113
laryngopharyngectomy, 61
laryngotracheal reconstruction (LTR), 116, 117

laryngo-tracheo-bronchoscopy (LTB), 88
laryngo-tracheo-oesophageal, 113
LeFort fractures, 154
Lemierre syndrome, 114
lentigo maligna, 133, 155
levobupivacaine, 176
lignocaine, 104
Lund-Mackay scores, 150
lymphatic drainage, 161

M

mandibulofacial dysostosis, 38
masking, 8, 32
maxillary nerve, 144
Meckel's cartilage, 103
melanoma, 158
Melkersson-Rosenthal syndrome, 71
MEN2A, 84
MEN2B, 85
Meniere's disease, 35, 39
methylprednisolone, 23
Michel deformity (complete labyrinthine aplasia), 47
microlaryngoscopy and bronchoscopy (MLB), 96, 97, 116, 118
microtia, 19
mitral stenosis, 57
Moraxella catarrhalis, 37
morphoeic BCC, 155
MRI internal auditory meati (MRI IAM), 5
mucoepidermoid carcinoma (MEC), 76–77
Muller manoeuvre, 63, 81
multidisciplinary team (MDT), 51, 124, 128, 137
multinodular thyroid goitre, 68, 73
Mustardé technique, 162–163
Mycoplasma pneumoniae, 39
myocardial infarction, 67
myringoplasty, 37

N

nasal endoscopy, 53
Naseptin therapy, 52
nasoethmoidal fractures, 162
nasopharyngeal cancer, 79
nasopharyngeal carcinoma (NPC), 52, 70
National Institute for Health and Care Excellence (NICE) guidance, 29, 61, 76, 78, 79
neck stiffness, 113

necrotising otitis externa (NOE), 22, 34, 34, 40, 40
neonatal intensive care unit (NICU), 28, 29, 87, 88
neonates, 102
newborn hearing screening programme in England (NHSP), 28
NF2-related schwannomatosis (NF2), 42–43
non-keratinising nasopharyngeal cancer, 61
non-steroidal antiinflammatory drugs (NSAIDs), 153
nystagmus, 11, 39

O

obstructive sleep apnoea (OSA), 58, 65, 75, 91, 120, 125
  adenotonsillectomy, 100
odynophagia, 96
oesophageal achalasia, 56, 74
ofloxacin, 29
oral candidiasis, 83
oral lichen planus (OLP), 52, 70, 85
oral ulceration, 65
orbital cellulitis, 146
organ of Corti, 28
orofacial granulomatosis, 71
Ortner's syndrome, 75
Osler-Weber-Rendu disease, 149
ossicular injury, 12
ossicular replacement prostheses, 30
ossiculoplasty, 21, 30
osteomeatal complex (OMC), 128, 148, 149
osteonecrosis, 15
otalgia, 1, 7
otitis, 7
otitis media with effusion (OME), 31
otoacoustic emissions (OAEs), 13, 24, 25
otological symptoms, 3
otomycosis, 6
otorrhoea, 1, 13
otosclerosis, 6–7, 30, 50
  bilateral, 8
otoscopy, 6, 14, 16

P

paediatric subglottic stenosis, 116
palatal myoclonus, 21
papillary thyroid cancer, 64
papillary thyroid carcinoma, 68
Paracusis of Willis, 28

paradoxical vocal cord dysfunction, 72
paraganglioma and pheochromocytoma (PGL/PCC) syndrome, 47
paragangliomas, 46
paramedian forehead flap (PMFF), 165
paranasal sinus, 156
parastomal recurrence, 85
parotid gland swelling, 58
partial ossicular replacement prostheses (PORPs), 12, 37
particle therapy, 69–70
Passavant's ridge, 117
Pearson correlation, 168, 175
pemphigus vulgaris (PV), 163
Pendred's syndrome, 48
pendred syndrome, 102
pentoxifylline, 33
peptic ulcer disease, 23
percutaneous tracheostomy, 62
perforated tympanic membrane, 13
perigeniculate facial nerve, 19
peritonsillar abscess, 114–115
permanent childhood hearing impairment (PCHI), 28
permanent threshold shift (PTS), 49
pharyngeal arches, 55
pharyngeal pouch, 51, 69
phonophobia, 15
Pierre Robin sequence (PRS), 88, 105
plain film radiography, 83
pleomorphic adenomas, 59, 76
Poiseuille's law, 96, 116
positron emission tomography-MRI (PET-MRI), 22
posterior septal perforations, 109
post-grommet infection, 121
Pott's puffy tumour, 144
presbycusis, 27, 29
processus cochleariformis, 22
profuse epistaxis, 170
prothrombin complex concentrate (PCC), 177
pseudomonas, 37
Pseudomonas aeruginosa, 22, 40
pulsatile tinnitus, 1, 21
pure tone audiogram (PTA), 24, 25, 45
purulent rhinorrhea, 93
p-value, 173

R

radical mastectomy, 17
radioactive iodine uptake (RIU), 76

radioallergosorbent (RAST), 171
radiologically inserted gastrostomy
    (RIG), 67
radiotherapy, 2
Ramsay-Hunt syndrome, 45
recurrent respiratory papillomatosis, 98, 118, 121
recurrent respiratory papillomatosis
    (RRP), 61
renal function tests, 83
respiratory papillomatosis, 98
retropharyngeal abscess, 115
retrosigmoid approach, 133–134
rheumatoid arthritis, 5, 57
rhinophyma, 162
rhinoscleroma, 146
rhytidectomy, 125
rigid bronchoscopy, 115
Rinne tuning fork tests, 16
Romberg's test, 11

S

Sadé grade 3 retraction, 16, 42
Sadé grade 4 retraction, 38, 42
salivary gland/duct caliculi, 75
Samter's triad, 153
sandifer syndrome (SS), 103
scapula, 56
Schaefer classification, 72
schwannomas, 44
sensorineural hearing loss (SNHL), 25, 49
septal perforation, 148, 152
septorhinoplasty, 125
severe sleep apnoea, 58
shortened columella, 161
sinonasal malignancies, 147
Sistrunk's procedure, 79–80
skin telangiectasia, 121
smoking cessation, 82
sofradex, 29
solitary median maxillary incisor syndrome, 103
sound localisation, 21, 23, 26
speech recognition threshold (SRT), 25
sphenopalatine artery, 126
spreader grafts, 145
squamous cell carcinoma (SCC), 40, 52, 56, 59, 69
    head and neck, 76
    hypopharyngeal, 60, 63
    hypopharynx extends, 78
    laryngectomy, 68
    ultraviolet (UV) radiation, 70

stapedial (acoustic) reflex testing, 45
stapes prosthesis, 7, 30
stapes superstructure, 7
Staphylococcus aureus, 37
steeple sign, 112
stereotactic radiosurgery, 46
sternocleidomastoid, 60, 68
Streptococcus pneumoniae, 9, 37, 39
Streptococcus pyogenes, 105
stylopharyngeus muscle, 65, 83
subglottic haemangiomas, 115
subglottic stenosis, 96
submandibular gland excision, 56
subtotal petrosectomy, 1
succinate dehydrogenase (SDH), 46
sulcus, 69
superficial parotidectomy, 63, 64
superior parathyroid glands, 54, 73
superior semicircular canal dehiscence
    syndrome (SSCDS), 36, 49–50, 168, 174
systemic steroids, 70

T

T1aN0M0 laryngeal cancer, 53
TCOF1 gene, 14
temporal bone trauma, 36
temporary threshold shift (TTS), 49
tensor tympani, 22, 22, 103
Thy3f/follicular lesion, 74
thymic aplasia, 88
thyroidectomy, 57, 63, 67
thyroid nodule, 59, 68
tinnitus, 19, 20
TMJ dysfunction, 13, 37
TNM staging, 53, 70
tonsillectomies, 92
tonsils, 77
total ossicular replacement prostheses
    (TORPs), 12, 33, 37
tracheoinnominate fistula (TIF), 79–80
tracheostomy, 97
tragal cartilage, 117
transient otoacoustic emissions (TOAEs), 38
translabyrinthine, 17, 46
Treacher Collins, 38
trephination, 157
trigeminal neuralgia, 72
trisomy 21, 8
Trypanosoma brucei, 74
Trypanosoma cruzi, 74
Tullio phenomenon, 35
12S ribosomal RNA gene, 24
tympanic membrane, 15

tympanic membrane retracts, 29
tympanic paraganglioma, 31
tympanograms, 4, 60
tympanomastoidectomy, 1, 9
tympanomastoid surgery, 2
tympanometry, 25, 25, 45, 50
tympanoplasty, 8, 13, 16, 37
type A tympanogram, 15
type II hypersensitivity, 179
type IV hypersensitivity, 179
type IV hypersensitivity, 38

U

unexplained vocal cord palsy, 64
unilateral hearing, 32
unilateral right-sided microtia, 8
University of Pennsylvania smell
        identification test (UPSIT), 132, 154
upper blepharoplasty, 162
upper respiratory tract infection, 2, 10, 14
urosepsis, 3
Usher's syndrome, 101, 111–112, 119, 121
uvulopalatopharyngoplasty (UVPP), 65

V

vagus nerves, 77
vascular endothelial growth factor (VEGF), 43

vasculitis/syphilis/Lyme disease, 35
vasomotor rhinitis, 152
vertical crest, 44
vertigo lasting, 11
vestibular evoked myogenic potentials
        (VEMPs), 41, 50, 168
vestibular neurectomy, 35
vestibular neuronitis, 35, 39
vestibular ocular reflex (VOR), 24
vidian artery, 157
visual analogue scale (VAS), 175
vitamin E, 33
vocal cord nodules, 69

W

Wallerian degeneration, 33–34,
        156
word recognition score (WRS), 25
Wullstein classification, 37

X

xylometazoline, 166, 171, 178

Z

Zenker's diverticulum, 69, 81
Z-plasty, 153

Printed in the United States
by Baker & Taylor Publisher Services

Printed in the United States
by Baker & Taylor Publisher Services